T0321193

Chinese Medicine for Health

Holistic Healing, Inner Harmony and Herbal Recipes

Chinese Medicine for Health

Holistic Healing, Inner Harmony and Herbal Recipes

Hong Hai

Renhai Centre Limited, Singapore &
Nanyang Technological University, Singapore

Karen Wee

Renhai Centre Limited, Singapore

Soh Shan Bin

Renhai Centre Limited, Singapore

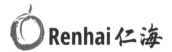 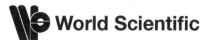

Published by

World Scientific Publishing Co. Pte. Ltd.

5 Toh Tuck Link, Singapore 596224

USA office: 27 Warren Street, Suite 401-402, Hackensack, NJ 07601

UK office: 57 Shelton Street, Covent Garden, London WC2H 9HE

Library of Congress Control Number: 2022940586

British Library Cataloguing-in-Publication Data
A catalogue record for this book is available from the British Library.

CHINESE MEDICINE FOR HEALTH
Holistic Healing, Inner Harmony and Herbal Recipes

ISBN 978-981-126-319-4 (hardcover)
ISBN 978-981-126-378-1 (paperback)
ISBN 978-981-126-320-0 (ebook for institutions)
ISBN 978-981-126-321-7 (ebook for individuals)

For any available supplementary material, please visit
https://www.worldscientific.com/worldscibooks/10.1142/13050#t=suppl

Typeset by Stallion Press
Email: enquiries@stallionpress.com

Printed in Singapore

"*Chinese Medicine for Health* is a rare find. Firstly, it is not easy to find a good TCM book written in English. Secondly, the authors have made the complexity and critical foundational concepts of TCM easy to understand and very readable. The *yangsheng* 养生 principles and delicious herbal recipes shared in the book will serve well seniors in their pursuit of total wellness and longevity."

Soh Swee Ping, Chief Executive Officer,
Council for Third Age (C3A)

"This is an extensively researched book on TCM written with great care and consideration, in clear and simple language. I especially like the chapter on *Yangsheng* (The Art of Cultivating Life), which is in line with Healthier SG in promoting wellness through physical, mental and spiritual health. The aim is to incorporate these principles into our lifestyle by combining Western ideas and Chinese wisdom into the art and science of living a balanced life. This should serve as our fundamental approach to health and disease prevention."

Dr Lily Aw, Senior Consultant Family Physician,
Fellow of the Academy of Medicine Singapore;
Registered Acupuncturist

"This comprehensive introductory book on Traditional Chinese Medicine (TCM) is commendable for its use of clear and simple language to explain TCM and interpret it in the context of Western medicine. It also distils ancient Chinese wisdom in the philosophy of TCM. An integral part of Chinese culture, TCM is more than an art of treatment. It also places emphasis on preventing disease and enhancing longevity. Western and Chinese Medicine practitioners should collaborate in research to develop a better system of medical care. Hopefully, this book will serve as a bridge between them."

Dr Koh Chin Aik, President,
Society of Traditional Chinese Medicine (Singapore)

"*Chinese Medicine for Health* is highly recommended for those who wish to have a better understanding of Traditional Chinese Medicine and for those who are looking for a holistic way to improve or maintain one's health. It is clear and concise, easy to read, captivating and include the authors' candid views on the future of Chinese Medicine. The reader will be inspired by the many easy-to-prepare recipes for tonics, preparations for various conditions as well as porridge, soups and herbal teas for cultivating life (*Yangsheng*)!"

Associate Professor Koh Hwee Ling, Dept of Pharmacy,
National University of Singapore

"This book is written with scintillating clarity. As a primer, it is the best available introductory book on Traditional Chinese Medicine. It covers a broad swath of the subject including history, philosophy, physiology, diet and preventive health. The quintessential elements of lifestyle in the Age Well Everyday program of the NUS Mind-Science Centre dovetail well with the ideas articulated by the authors.

It is as absorbing and piquing as its companion volume, *Principles of Chinese Medicine: A Modern Interpretation*."

Professor Kua Ee Heok,
Tan Geok Yin Professor in Psychiatry & Neuroscience,
National University of Singapore

"If you are looking for ways to have a healthy life you will be rewarded to read and practise the gems expounded in this book. The authors succinctly explain the basics of TCM, dispensed in just the right doses. Concepts of causes, diagnosis and treatment of illnesses are clearly explained. While there is some mention of contraindications of TCM treatments, this important subject calls for more specialised research, albeit outside the scope of this introductory book.

For those interested in eating like an emperor, chapters 13 and 14 on *"yangsheng"* are must reads. Enjoy good health and beauty!"

Dr Tan Chay Hoon, President,
Asia College of Neuropsychopharmacology,
Honorary Fellow and former Associate Professor of Pharmacology,
National University of Singapore

Functional or integrative medicine, popularised in the 1990s, centres around a holistic, personalised approach to health and healing. *Chinese Medicine for Health* shows me that TCM fundamentally adopts this philosophy! The patient-centric approach of TCM and its important concept of *yangsheng* are clearly and simply explained.

The authors have dissected the complexities of the ancient Chinese medical classic *Huangdi Neijing* in a comprehensive yet easily comprehensible manner for ordinary folks.

Genevieve Chua, Chief Executive Officer,
OVOL Singapore Pte Ltd

Chinese medicine has brought healing and good health to millions through the ages. Because of its close link to the Chinese culture, however, it can seem abstruse to those who do not know the language. This new book demystifies the art and science of Chinese medicine. With sound knowledge of both Western and Chinese medicine, the authors have produced the finest English exposition yet of Chinese medicine. *Chinese Medicine for Health* is a must-read for medical professionals as well as anyone simply wishing to live healthier and longer.

Dr Michael Tai, Fellow of the Royal Asiatic Society of Great Britain and Ireland

"*Chinese Medicine for Health* is everyone's guide to achieving and maintaining a positive integration of Mind, Body and Spirit. It is a compendium of the wisdom of ancient Chinese medicine and practices for *yangsheng*. The authors explain TCM concepts in a highly approachable style. I particularly like the detailed descriptions of herbs, acupuncture, recipes for soups, tonics and teas. This book is a valuable resource for anyone interested in pursuing a fulfilling life in health and wellbeing."

Carmee Lee, Mentor Principal, MindChamps Holdings;
Founder & President, Aoede Music Enterprise Pte Ltd

"A fascinating book from the perspective of a lay person. The recipes are very informative and useful. Porridge is in our daily diet but until I read the book, I had never realized that it can be for *yangsheng* too!"

Dr Lee Chay Hoon, Director,
Organization Development and Human Resource,
Keppel Offshore and Marine

Preface

Chinese medicine, an ancient art and science of more than five thousand years, has shown surprising resilience in the face of dazzling advances in modern biomedical medicine. Today, Chinese medical clinics continue to thrive not only in their traditional base in the East, but also in the West where, ironically, technological advances in biomedicine leave a wide gap for holistic naturalistic methods of healing to fill.

We published *Pursuing the Elixir of Life: Chinese Medicine for Health* in 2016 as a textbook for traditional Chinese medicine (TCM) courses run by us. We have been encouraged by generations of course participants taking zealously to Chinese medicine for improving their health and those of their loved ones. After several reprints and positive feedback received from readers, we felt it was time to rewrite the book as a general introduction to Chinese medicine, with a heavier emphasis on the use of medicinal herbs for improving personal health.

This new book offers simplified explanations of the theoretical principles of Chinese medicine before introducing readers to methods of diagnosis and treatment, acupuncture, management of chronic illnesses, and *yangsheng* (the cultivation of life). Much of the rest of the book is devoted to herbs and formulations, including over a hundred medicated food and tea recipes on which readers can try their culinary skills. Readers who are less interested in TCM theory may skip chapters 2 and 4 on a first reading of the book.

Traditional Chinese medical principles are difficult to explain because much of it appears to be at variance with biomedical science. We have explained Chinese medical theory in a new and novel way, so that people with a basic knowledge of science can relate to its concepts and methods and apply them to diet, therapies, and the cultivation of health.

The therapeutic value of Chinese medical formulations has rarely been accepted by modern mainstream biomedical science. As practioners of TCM, we have little doubt about their safety and efficacy. Nevertheless, we make the disclaimer that most of the therapies described in this book have not undergone large-scale randomized controlled clinical trials that are the standard fare of evidence-based medicine backed by pharmaceutical companies with large resources. As argued in the final chapter of the book, there is no financial incentive for commercial pharmaceutical companies to run costly trials on ancient formulations for which no patents can be claimed. However numerous small-scale clinical trials can be found in the scientific literature, as well as voluminous clinical records and case studies in TCM clinics around the world.

We hope that readers will enjoy reading the book and learning practical ways to improve their health through the wisdom of holistic and natural methods in Chinese medicine.

This book can be read with Hong Hai's *Principles of Chinese Medicine: A Modern Interpretation* which treats the theory of Chinese medicine in greater depth and explains the scientific and philosophical foundations of TCM.

We thank Joy Fang, senior editor at World Scientific Publishing Company for her professionalism and tireless effort in bringing this book to print, and our many readers and supporters.

Hong Hai
Karen Wee Yan Ling
Soh Shan Bin
of The Renhai Clinic

Contents

List of Recipes

I. Recipes for Therapy

II. *Yangsheng foods and teas*

Chapter 1

Introduction: The Origins and Significance of Chinese Medicine

Traditional Chinese medicine (TCM) is both an art and a science.

It is an art in that there is a great deal of personal judgment involved in Chinese medical healing. Diagnosis and prescribed therapy take account of not only the clinical signs shown by the patient, but also their physical environment, emotional state and social connections with family and community.

TCM is a science in the sense that the rules of diagnosis and therapy were developed from empirical experience. It is the distillation of thousands of years of case studies as well as, in modern times, small to medium scale clinical trials on herbal remedies, acupuncture, tuina and qigong exercises.

Chinese medicine is not just a method of healing. It is a culture of living a full life with good health and finding fulfilment in harmony with nature and society.

Chinese medicine is widespread not only in East Asia, where it has a long history, but also in the developed countries of the West. What is special about Chinese medicine that makes it a mystery to most Western biomedical scientists, yet passionately embraced by myriads of users worldwide? The answer most likely lies in its efficacy in promoting health and treating illnesses.

Chinese medicine's enduring popularity derives from its roots in both medical and social sciences. It is steeped in ancient culture and philosophy backed by the clinical experience of hundreds of generations of physicians dedicated to conquering illness and promoting health. Many of the ideas in TCM may be found in Chinese literature and ancient philosophical writings.

In Singapore, approximately forty percent of visits to licensed medical practitioners are to Chinese medical clinics. Chinese medicine and locally adapted versions of it are practised extensively in Asian countries from China through Korea and Vietnam to Indonesia. It also has many loyal adherents in Western societies of Australia, Britain, Europe, and the Americas.

1.1 Medicine in Chinese Society

Chinese medicine was a gem of Chinese science. It was an integral part of the Chinese culture, closely knit with its language and cuisine, permeating the daily lives of Mandarins and commoners alike. A Chinese person would speak of "internal heat", not to mean a fever in the body, but the condition of a sore throat, ruddy face, quick pulse and yellow tinge on the fur of the tongue. A bitter concoction of heat clearing herbs would readily be administered and most of the time the symptoms would resolve.

The use of herbal ingredients in food was essential knowledge for mothers, who would add tonics like astragalus and Chinese yam to soups if they saw signs of weak qi in their children. They might use herbs like ginseng and *duzhong* (eucommia bark) to enhance the growth of sinews and bones.

So pervasive was the culture of Chinese medicine that the exquisite herbal recipes used by the gentry in the great Qing classic *Hongloumeng* (*Dream of the Red Chamber*) have spawned dozens of scholarly works in modern times devoted to the study of their culinary and medical genius.

Until the second half of the 20th century, Chinese medicine was the main system of health and healing in China, faithfully serving emperors and concubines in palaces, soldiers in battlefield, and humble folks in farms and city streets. Well into the 21st century, traditional Chinese medicine (TCM) remains the most significant alternative to modern Western ("biomedicine") in the industrialized economies. In many areas of medicine that have enjoyed the best of modern biomedical technology, TCM continues to find a unique role.

For example, in the cardiology department of the Guang'anmen Hospital of the China Academy of Chinese Medical Science in Beijing, one group of patients with ischemic heart disease have previously received series of stents in other hospitals, but many see their arteries continue to clog up despite large doses of statins and anti-coagulant drugs. They were administered herbal formulations containing such ingredients as ginseng, *chuanxiong* and safflower to reduce the incidence of further blockages.

In the 2002 global outbreak of the severe acute respiratory syndrome (SARS), the average mortality rate in China was 7% compared to 12%–25% in the other countries. Only China combined TCM herbs with Western therapies that used steroids and antipyretics.[1] In more recent times, Chinese remedies have been found to help in the recovery of patients afflicted by the Covid-19 virus.[2]

Faith in Chinese medicine is growing in Western countries. At the Cleveland Clinic in the United States, a TCM department was set up in 2014.[3] Clinic administrators stated that while clinical trials of the efficacy of Chinese medical treatments were ongoing, patients felt they were getting better with these treatments and kept coming back for more. The clinic's current website states, "There is a growing body of evidence supporting Chinese herbal therapy for many acute and chronic conditions."[4]

---

[1] World Health Organisation (2004)
[2] Myn Lyu *et al* (2021)
[3] *Wall Street Journal* (2014)
[4] Cleveland Clinic (2022)

1.2 Medicine in Ancient China

Chinese medicine has origins going back several millennia to herbalists like Shen Nong (*circa* 2500 BC) who collected leaves, roots and animal parts that had healing powers. Shen Nong painstakingly recorded the effects of these herbs on his patients. He even tried many herbs on himself, such was his devotion to empirical evidence. Legend has it that he eventually died from poisoning by one of the herbs, but not before he had recorded 365 herbs and their characteristics in the first formal pharmacopeia of Chinese medicine, *Shen Nong Ben Cao Jing* (神农本草经).

The early practitioners of acupuncture used sharpened stones to exert pressure on selected points in the body and discovered that this could ease pain and promote flows in the body to achieve internal balance and healing. This laid the foundation of the complex science of acupuncture, now practised in modern clinics throughout the world and approved for health insurance claims in many countries.

Chinese medicine was not always based on science. In antiquity, healing was commonly attributed to pacifying the spirits. It was believed that people fell ill because they were possessed by evil spirits and demons. Mediums had to be employed to pray and appease or drive away these spirits. There were similar practices in Greece and Rome in the form of temple medicine. Sick people would sleep in temples in the belief that in their dreams the gods would appear to chase away the spirits that troubled them.

As physicians studied medical cases of patients and handed down their accumulated knowledge and wisdom, the observations and conclusions of empirical science gained dominance. Careful records of eminent physicians of the Han dynasty (206BC-220AD) were compiled in the first and greatest of all Chinese medical classics, the *Huangdi Neijing* (黄帝内经).

The *Neijing* declared that illnesses were not caused by spiritual agents but by natural forces, comprising climatic, dietary, lifestyle and emotional influences. Over the next 2000 years, hundreds of noted physicians further developed and refined these ideas into the Chinese medicine taught today in medical colleges and practised in clinics all over the world.

1.3 Chinese Medicine in Modern Times

Up to the first half of the 20th century, Chinese medicine was mainstream medicine, but its position was increasingly challenged by scholars who had studied Western medicine abroad after the May 4th Movement (五四运动) of 1919, which marked the beginning of the modernisation of China. Returned scholars were determined to change China by introducing science and technology. One of the consequences of this movement was that the scientific nature of Chinese medicine came into question. Some Western educated physicians, confident of the superiority of their newfound knowledge, urged the government to phase out Chinese medicine and replace it with Western medicine. Several decades of debate and contention followed. The issue was not settled until the ascendancy of Chairman Mao Zedong after the 1949 Chinese Revolution.

Mao was a believer of Chinese medicine, calling it a "a treasure trove of Chinese wisdom," but felt that Chinese medicine had to be modernised by absorbing some of the ideas and methods of Western medicine. One result of this was that some of the nation's best Chinese medical scholars were tasked to record and systematise medical knowledge into textbooks similar to those used in Western medical schools.

Although the intervention of Mao's new government helped to preserve Chinese medicine, the ancient science had to compete against the vaunted efficacy of Western medicine backed by giant pharmaceutical companies with deep pockets for research. Chinese medicine survived and thrived only because patients were getting well after receiving treatment. In many instances of chronic disorders like skin eczema, digestive problems, menstrual issues, menopausal syndrome, persistent dry cough and back pain, Chinese medicine offers effective remedies that encourage many patients to seek TCM treatment over Western therapies.

From the 1960s, medical training was carried out through new colleges of Chinese medicine offering undergraduate and post-graduate degrees. Chinese medicine taught formally and practised this way became known as "Traditional Chinese Medicine" (TCM). In China and Taiwan today, Chinese and Western medicine are practised side by side in many major hospitals and clinics. In a real way, their patients enjoy the best of both worlds.

It should be noted that TCM taught and practised under government regulatory supervision is different from a variety of old Chinese practices not incorporated in modern textbooks. The latter may be classified as folk medicine. They use methods that do not fall within mainstream of Chinese medicine and are not recognised for practice by physicians holding practising licenses from health authorities in China, Hong Kong, Taiwan, Malaysia and Singapore.

Chapter 2

Basic Substances in the Human Body

When learning Chinese medicine, we need to temporarily put aside modern knowledge of human physiology.

Instead, we need to view ancient models of the human body as an alternative way of characterizing human physiology for purposes of diagnosis and treatment of illnesses and finding ways to achieve good health. These models have proven, over thousands of years, to be useful in curing disease and enhancing health, and should be taken at face value as practical and useful models that historically have produced good results. The test of the pudding, as the saying goes, is in the eating.

The ancients simplified human anatomy and physiology to fundamental building blocks that fitted their view of the workings of the body. Among these building blocks is the notion that there are fundamental substances or ingredients of the body that are involved in all physiological processes. To have these ingredients in sufficient quantity and functioning smoothly in the body is thus an important basis of wellness.

The basic ingredients are qi (气), blood or *xue* (血), and essence or *jing* (精), as well as clear body fluids known as *jinye* (津液). The first three are collectively known as the three precious ingredients, or *sanbao* (三宝) as they are essential to human vitality and should be carefully cultivated and preserved as though they are treasures in the human body.

Of these, qi is the most widely observed, present in almost every physiological process in the body. Lack of qi or hindrances to its smooth flow in the body spells health problems.

How did qi come to be so important and powerful a concept in Chinese medicine? Qi indeed has a history as old as Chinese civilization. Its mythical origins go back to the beginning of time in Chinese cosmology.

2.1 Qi 气

In Chinese cosmology qi from early antiquity was regarded as the most basic constituent of the universe. At the birth of the universe, qi was the origin of all substances, processes and energy forces. Because of these ancient Chinese beliefs, the word "qi" found its way into numerous uses in the Chinese language to describe concepts involving flow, movement, or energy. For example, *qixiang* (气象) means weather. *Qizhi* (气质) refers to the innate quality of your personality, and *qise* (气色) the glow of health on your face. Qi is used even to describe the tone and spirit of a literary work, as in *qiyun* (气韵).

Qi was naturally adopted into Chinese medical theory, and over time it acquired definite technical meanings in the vocabulary of Chinese physicians. In Chinese medicine, qi has a special meaning and should not be confused with its numerous applications in everyday language, even if they have common historical origins. In TCM language, qi has two aspects. It is a kind of vital force driving flow and change in the body. It is also a kind of substance that stores the energy of the vital force.

One might legitimately ask: is qi a form of energy, or is it a substance? The answer is that it is both. Ancient Chinese philosophy did not rigidly distinguish between energy and material substances. One can make the interesting argument that this insight of ancient Chinese thinkers presaged the revolutionary discovery in Albert Einstein's general theory of relativity. Einstein showed that mass (material) and energy can be converted into each other. In modern living, it has become common to see mass converted to energy in a nuclear reactor, or an atomic bomb explosion.[5]

Forms of qi

There are many kinds of qi. Qi can also be classified by its role in the body, or by where it is located.

Thus *weiqi* (卫气) is defensive armour at the outer layers of the body which prevents the invasion of harmful influences known as pathogens. *Yingqi* (营气) is nutrient qi that circulates and nourishes the body.

Qi in the lower abdomen area prevents prolapse of the lower organs, and qi in the skin prevents excessive sweating.

Zongqi (宗气) refers to the pectoral qi that, according to ancient understanding, resides below the sternum (breastbone), akin to a reservoir of special energy that allows one to have a sonorous voice. A good singer would be regarded as having good *zongqi*. As a practical matter, in modern biological terms, when we say that a man has strong *zongqi*, we mean that his lung and diaphragm muscles are strong, his respiratory tracts are clear, his vocal cords in good tone, and there is sufficient blood circulation to energize the relevant muscles. Thus, having good *zongqi* is TCM's way of saying one has this excellent voice capability.

This example illustrates to us an important point about TCM concepts. TCM often uses analogy to convey meaning. Saying that the person has a good reservoir of *zongqi* below his breastbone is a graphic way of saying he has all those physiological conditions to produce an admirable voice quality.

The example also highlights the importance of regarding TCM terms like qi as denoting a certain capability and not necessarily any

---

[5] Mass is converted to energy by the classic formula the classic equation $E = mc^2$, where E is energy, m is mass and c is the speed of light.

identifiable substance or energy source with measurable properties. Likewise, as we shall see later in the book, the concept of "dampness" does not refer to high humidity, but instead to an internal condition which makes a person feel lethargy and digestive discomfort. We hope the reader keeps this point constantly in mind when learning TCM. It is a common source of perplexity when you cannot relate a TCM term to the usage of the same word in daily life. We should therefore be vigilant when using TCM special terms to differentiate them from their meanings in non-medical usage.

In general, any physiological activity has some form of qi behind it. Qi can be imagined as a kind of a vital force for maintaining life activities, driving the functions of the organs and meridians. Thus, we speak of spleen qi, kidney qi, heart qi and other forms of qi that are involved in the functions of these organs. Qi that is stored in the organs can be conceptualized as a form of stored energy, to be converted into energy when needed.

From where does the body get its qi? Qi is acquired in several ways. Through our parents, we are born with congenital qi or *yuanqi* (元气) stored in the kidney. *Yuanqi* is also known as primordial qi or original qi. The amount of *yuanqi* inherited from parents affects the health and development of the baby. After birth, we acquire more qi from food, exercise, and air from breathing. Blood is also involved in the production of qi. The spleen, which governs digestion, transforms food into nutrients which combine with air to form qi.

The functions of qi

Another way of understanding qi is to look at its functions. There are broadly five functions.

1. Driving function. Qi drives, or propels, the functions of all the organs of the body. For example, heart qi drives blood circulation;

in the spleen qi promotes digestion and absorption of food; lung qi governs respiration.

2. Warming function. Qi warms the body and is the source of heat energy and plays a key role in maintaining normal body temperature.

3. Defensive function. Healthy qi protects the body by resisting the invasion of harmful pathogens.

4. Controlling function. Qi plays a role in controlling blood and body fluids, to prevent them from leaking or unduly flowing out of the body. In the case of blood, qi keeps it flowing inside the blood capillaries and prevents it from oozing out into the surrounding tissue. Failure to control body fluids may result in urinary incontinence or excessive salivation.

5. Transforming function. This function is very wide, and includes transforming external nutrients into blood, qi, essence, and body fluids. Waste substances and turbid qi are also excreted from the body.

In summary, qi is involved in all physiological processes in the body. It drives flow and movement, transforms external materials into nutrients, transforms one basic ingredient of life into another, excretes waste from the body, and protects the body from harmful environmental factors. It is no wonder that qi is also known as the "root of life" (生命之根本).

A note on *Zhengqi* or healthy qi

Another use of the term qi is *zhengqi* (正气). This is strictly speaking not a particular form of qi. Instead, it is an over-arching concept that denotes the overall capability of the body to carry out its physiological functions smoothly and efficiently, and to fight against invasions of harmful pathogens. *Zhengqi* is also known as healthy qi, vital qi, and genuine qi. Western interpretations of *zhengqi* sometimes liken it to the body's immune system. It is a good analogy, but somewhat incomplete as *zhengqi* more than protects. Its abundance indicates the healthy functioning of the body.

Hence, to say that the body has adequate *zhengqi* is just another way of saying that it is functioning in an efficient and healthy manner. That is why the *Huangdi Neijing* has a famous aphorism, "*Zhengqi nei cun, xie buke gan*" (正气内存，邪不可干), which means that if the body has adequate healthy qi, pathogens cannot take hold.

2.2 Blood 血

In TCM, blood or *xue* (血) has a wider meaning than the same term used in modern physiology. In Chinese medicine, blood has three main functions.

Functions of blood

1. Nourishing and moistening. Circulating to every part of the body, blood nourishes and moistens to enable each part of the body to perform life's activities. When there is sufficient blood, the organs get good nourishment, and the person may have a ruddy and glowing complexion, lustrous hair and skin, and strong muscles. If blood is deficient, the person has a pale complexion and may suffer from dizziness, hair loss, dry rough skin, numbness of limbs and, in the case of women, menstrual issues.
2. Enables mental activities. Blood fuels mental activities such as concentration and sound sleep. A person who is deficient in blood may suffer from insomnia and forgetfulness.
3. Excretion. Blood transports turbid (used) qi to the lung for excretion through respiration. It also transports waste materials for excretion to the kidney through urine, and to the skin through perspiration.

Circulation and production of blood

The physiology of blood circulation and production in TCM is significantly different from that of blood in modern physiology.

In TCM, the main driver of blood circulation is the propelling function of heart qi. Hence a deficiency in qi can lead to poor blood circulation.

In addition, the lung, spleen and liver also play important roles in blood circulation. The lung is connected with many large vessels and helps in propelling qi and blood flow. Spleen qi enables blood to stay within the capillaries. The liver stores blood and regulates the volume of blood in circulation that is appropriate for the body's activities at any time.

Hence good blood circulation requires the coordination and cooperation of the heart, lung, spleen and liver. TCM thus views blood circulation holistically, involving five main organs as well as the propelling function of qi.

We find a similar holistic explanation for the production of blood. As in blood circulation, the spleen, stomach, heart, lung, and liver each play a role in blood production.

There are two major sources of blood. Food ingested by the body is converted to many products including nutrient qi, which then combines with body fluid to form blood.

Blood can also be formed by conversion from *jing* (essence) in the kidney. As we shall see below, essence is stored in the kidney. Hence the kidney plays a role in producing blood by supplying the liver with essence for conversion.

Relationship between blood and qi

The circulation of blood is propelled by the heart using heart qi. In addition, qi is involved in the production of blood, and blood is involved in the production of qi.

Qi and blood are thus closely related, like a pair of inseparable twins. Their close relationship is described in the lively analogy, "Qi is the marshal of blood and blood is the mother of qi." (气为血之帅, 血为气之母).

Qi is the marshal of blood because qi promotes the flow of blood. Without qi as the driving force, flow of blood is stagnated and blood cannot be efficiently transported to all parts of the body. Furthermore, qi participates in the production of blood, and enables blood to stay within the blood vessels instead. Therefore, a person who is qi-deficient may also be vulnerable to internal bleeding.

On the other hand, blood is the mother of qi. This is because blood nourishes and carries qi to assist in its circulation. When qi accompanied by blood, it moves along correct paths without being dispersed. This explains why when someone suffers from severe haemorrhage there is a loss of not only blood but also qi.

Blood and qi are like two sides of a coin. One cannot not exist without the other.

2.3 Body Fluids 津液

Another important entity in our body is body fluids (*jinye* 津液). We know in practice there are hundreds of kinds of body fluids in our body such as hormonal secretions, digestive juices etc. But in the Chinese model, everything is included under the umbrella of *jinye*.

The scope of *jinye* is very wide and it has many functions of the various body fluids and secretions found in modern physiology.

Like qi and blood, *jinye* is produced from food by the organs. The thin body fluids are usually found in muscles, skin and orifices whereas the thick body fluids are found in the organs and marrow. Its main functions are to nourish, participate in blood production and transport turbid qi.

2.4 *Jing* 精 or Essence

The body also has a more esoteric substance known as essence or *jing* (精) that we do not hear about as often as qi, blood, and body fluids in connection with TCM diagnosis and treatment. Nevertheless, it is useful to cover essence briefly as you may occasionally come across it in Chinese medical literature.

There are two kinds of essence — innate essence and acquired essence.

Innate essence (先天之精) is stored in the kidney and inherited from parents, carrying with it the inherited characteristics of the parents. Innate essence has commonality with genes in biomedical science. Like genes, innate essence endows a child with the biological characteristics of both parents.

One form of innate essence is male semen, which contains sperms that carry the characteristics of the father that are passed on to the child.

Acquired essence (后天之精) refers to refined nutritious substances transformed by qi from food. It enables life activities, nourishing all the organs.

The combination of innate and acquired essences produces kidney qi, which is involved in reproduction of offspring and in growth and development of children.

Essence is closely related to qi. Essence is a source of qi, as it can be converted to qi. Conversely, qi can be used to replenish essence.

The relationship between qi and essence is so close that one sometimes refers to them as one compound entity, *jingqi* (精气).

Chapter 3

Distinguishing Aspects of TCM

Several features of TCM distinguish it from Western medicine. These may be broadly divided into two categories:

a. the holistic character of TCM
b. their unique way of looking at the causes and remedies for illnesses through the concept of "syndromes"

The holistic nature of TCM views the human body as healthy when it enjoys internal harmony, which also requires harmony with nature. This implies that one should look for the disharmonies when a person falls ill. Treatment then aims at eliminating the disharmonies, not just at reducing the symptoms of the illness.

TCM uses the unique concept of syndromes to identify and classify the disharmonies. The diagnosis of illness thus consists of identifying the syndrome and treating the syndrome accordingly. This is known formally as "differentiating the syndrome and treating the patient accordingly," or *bian zheng lun zhi* (辨证论治).

3.1 Holism and Harmony

The concept of holism is central to Chinese medical philosophy. Holism, as the term implies, means viewing things as a whole rather than in parts. It requires seeing the big picture and regarding the body as a functioning organism with all its parts working together in harmony and in accordance with regularities of nature.

In his celebrated verse on the majestic Mount Lu (*Lushan*), the renowned poet Su Dongpo declared,

I do not know the true face of Lushan,
But only because I am in the midst of the mountain.
不知庐山真面目,
只缘身在此山中.

When you are inside the mountain, you can only see the foliage, tree trunks, and green undergrowth, but you have no idea what the whole mountain actually looks like. To view the mountain, you have to look at it from a distance to appreciate its beauty and its relation to the environment.

Likewise, if you look only at the part of the body that feels unwell, you merely have an incomplete understanding of its condition. If you look only at the cells and genes that are the building blocks of the body, you would fail to understand the workings of the body as a whole. For example, if your stomach feels discomfort and doctors look only at the stomach lining through an endoscope and do not observe important symptoms like lassitude, aversion to cold or nervous tension that are related to the stomach disorder, they would have only a limited understanding of your condition.

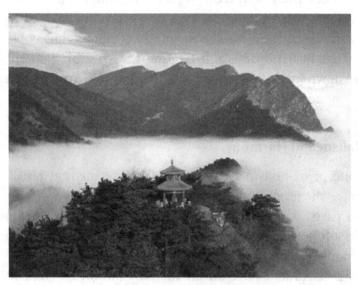

Fig. 3.1   Lushan in Jiangxi province

Of course, Western medicine also looks at the body as a whole. But there is the attraction of technology that allows observation of disease at the microscopic level, a capability that reflects the attitude of "reductionist medicine." This may tend to distract the physician from a holistic view of the condition.

This reductionist emphasis has been influenced by reductionism in the physical sciences. But even the genius of modern physics Albert Einstein once lamented, "Many scientists...seem to be like somebody who has seen thousands of trees but has never seen a forest."

In ancient times, Chinese physicians did not have microscopes, electronic scans, and laboratories to examine tissue, cells, and blood. They could only look at the body's external manifestations. Hence Chinese diagnosis and therapies were naturally focussed on the body as a whole and sought explanations for illnesses accordingly.

The holism approach may be expressed as defining health to be a state when the body achieves internal harmony. When there is harmony, there is internal balance, and the body enjoys smooth flows of qi, blood and other fluids.

Balance

When the body has internal balance, there is no deficiency or excess of yin and yang. There is also no deficiency of qi, essence, blood, or body fluids.

Yin is cool and moist; yang is warm and dry. When yin is deficient, the body is dry and warm, which can be felt in the mouth, eyes, skin and lungs. Yin deficiency of the kidney and liver causes dryness in the eyes, throat and other parts of the body. The person feels warm and vexatious, and there can be hot flashes, as happens commonly to menopausal women. Western treatment by hormonal replacement therapy for such menopausal symptoms may have side effects. TCM treats more conservatively by nourishing yin with tonics such as *Liuwei Dihuang Wan* (六味地黄丸).

When yang is deficient, the body is afraid of cold, and there may be back pain, tiredness and, in the case of men, sexual dysfunction. Yang tonic formulations such as *Shenqiwan* (肾气丸) may be helpful.

(Yin and yang will be explained in more detail in the next chapter.)

Flows

Smooth flow of qi, blood and body fluids is essential to the normal functioning of the organs. Lack of flow is associated with pain, hence the aphorism "When there is no flow, there is pain; when there is no pain, there is flow" (不通则痛，不痛则通). This means that the source of pain is poor flow. Qi stagnation, blood stasis, dampness and phlegm are forms of impeded flows of one kind or another. They are the underlying causes of many illnesses.

For example, Chinese medicine attributes arthritic pain of the joints to qi or blood not flowing properly. This results in inflammation, as wear and tear in the body has not been repaired and cleared up properly. To treat arthritic pain, we should promote flow of blood and qi to reduce the flow impediments that cause inflammation. The use of painkillers or anti-inflammatory drugs like steroids and NSAIDs only provide symptomatic relief.

Coronary heart disease, strokes and vascular dementia may also be viewed in terms of poor flow of qi and blood that results in blockages. TCM remedies attempt to improve these flows with qi tonics and formulations that improve blood flow and reduce a kind of blood flow impediment that TCM calls blood stasis (*yuxue* 瘀血). We shall have more to say about blood stasis in later chapters of the book.

3.2 Syndromes

The TCM concept of syndromes is unique and holds the key to understanding the Chinese approach to the diagnosis and treatment of illnesses. Furthermore, the prevention of syndromes underlies the Chinese approach to health cultivation and the prevention of illness.

It is important to emphasize that the term syndrome in Chinese medicine is distinct and different from the same term in Western medical usage for conditions like Down's syndrome. A TCM syndrome (*zheng* 证) is a collection of symptoms with an identifiable pattern.

A common example of a TCM syndrome is "heat" (*re* 热), which should be understood differently from heat that causes substances to rise in temperature and feel hot, or the body to run a fever. When you have a TCM heat syndrome (and the body is said in local slang to be "heaty"), it means that you have symptoms like a dry throat and a feeling of vexatiousness. There may be a yellow coating (fur) on the tongue; the pulse is faster than normal. The body temperature may well be normal.

Later this book, we shall come across many other syndromes, like dampness, wind, yin deficiency, qi deficiency, and qi or blood stagnation. Such syndromes define the body conditions diagnosed by TCM methods. Each condition is a health disorder or illness that needs to be treated by TCM methods for resolving syndromes. Often a patient presents more than one syndrome. For example, they may have both heat and dampness, and are then said to suffer from the compound syndrome of heat dampness.

Diagnosis of illness is mostly a matter of identifying the syndrome(s) present in the body. Treatment consists of resolving the syndromes. For example, arthritic pain may be due to poor flow of qi and blood and internal dampness. Treatment can be by herbs and qigong exercise to promote qi and blood flow and remove dampness. For many who seek TCM treatment, these may provide longer term relief than synthetic anti-inflammatory drugs.

TCM is patient-centric

TCM is patient-centric in the sense that it focusses on the underlying condition of the individual person's body, including their state of mind and social environment, rather than on the disease itself. This is because the same disease may be caused by different syndromes, and treatment must be according to the underlying syndrome. Conversely, different diseases may have the same underlying syndrome, in which case the same treatment can be applied to both. This is the rationale behind the important saying in Chinese medicine, "Same disease, different treatments; different diseases, same treatment" (同病异治; 异病同治).

An example of "same disease different treatments" is chronic headache. This can be from internal heat, or it can arise from qi deficiency resulting in insufficient qi and blood flow to the head. In the former case, treatment is by eliminating internal heat with suitable herbs or acupuncture. In the latter case, application of appropriate qi tonics may resolve the problem. Modern painkiller drugs provide symptomatic relief, but do not resolve the underlying syndromes.

An example of the same treatment applied to different disease conditions is smoothing the flow of liver qi (*shugan* 疏肝) to overcome qi stagnation. Liver qi stagnation can cause digestive problems like acid reflux and bloatedness. It can also cause insomnia. The herbs *chaihu* (柴胡) and *shaoyao* (芍药) are commonly used together in formulations to resolve digestive problems as well as insomnia due to liver qi stagnation.

The renowned Canadian physician William Osler, who helped found John Hopkins Medical School and was the Oxford Regius Professor of medicine, was known to be a discerning patient-centric healer. Osler famously said, "The good physician treats the disease; the great physician treats the patient who has the disease."[6] He would have found hearty approval from TCM physicians.

Prevention over Cure

Although both Chinese and Western medicine place emphasis on prevention of illness, TCM has the added feature of preventing

---

[6] Life in the Fastlane (2022)

subclinical illness (*ya jian kang* 亚健康) before they develop into clinical illness. For example, a man may have a dry throat, feel vexatious and show a red tongue with little fur. A TCM diagnosis indicates he has yin deficiency of the lung. However, a Western doctor would not normally detect an illness, as listening to his lungs through a stethoscope or examining his blood would not reveal any pathology. There are no known biomarkers for lung yin deficiency. To the TCM physician, this is an imbalance, an early stage of an illness. If left untreated, the patient could develop a persistent dry cough that is hard to resolve.

The World Health Organisation has estimated that about 70% of the world population is in the subclinical illness category. They will develop more serious illnesses later if the conditions are left untreated. TCM diagnosis can pick up subclinical illnesses through syndrome differentiation and nip the problems in the bud.

In traditional China, family physicians were rewarded with better bonuses each year if they dispensed very little medicine during the year to treat illnesses. They had prevented mild syndromes from developing into diseases that required strong medications. Instead, they used diet, herbal tonics and other mild prophylactic concoctions to keep family healthy. They also inculcated good living habits in the family to prevent serious conditions from developing. This is called *zhi weibing* (治未病) or curing an illness before it develops clinical symptoms. It is one of the unique and enduring strengths of Chinese medicine.

Chapter 4

Yin Yang, Five Elements
and TCM Organs

Chinese medicine views the human body in terms of relationships among vital organs and the role of the basic substances like qi and blood in the functioning of organs. Such a view enables working models for diagnosis and treatment of illnesses to incorporate the accumulated experience of physicians over the ages.

These models were inspired by ancient philosophy and cosmology, which saw the inner universe within the body to be a microcosm, a miniature replica, of the outer universe. They looked to certain regularities observed in nature and tried to see similar patterns within the human body.

As a practical matter, physicians had to contend with human illness and sought models of the workings of the human body that would guide them in healing the sick. The result was a set of principles that best fit their clinical experience. These principles were refined over hundreds of years into the narrative of the *Huangdi Neijing*, which expounds a system of medicine that has stood the test of time.

We describe below two of the fundamental models of the human body's inner workings: the Yin-Yang Principle and the Five-Element Model. Although historically derived from ancient cosmology, in medicine they are empirically based models for practical use and do not have cosmological or spiritual implications. Although we shall touch on the scientific rationale for these models, a more thorough treatment is outside the scope of this book and must be left to a more advanced theoretical text.[7] In this chapter we explain how these models work, and the intriguing ways in which they help in medical diagnosis and therapy.

4.1 The Yin-Yang Principle

The concept of yin and yang is fundamental to Chinese culture. It draws on observations of dualism in nature, in which entities and attributes tend to exist in pairs – male and female, soft and hard, night and day. These are relationships and interactions between two contrasting entities that capture the profound meaning of harmony and balance not just in the natural world but also in human and societal relationships. The wisdom of the yin and yang principle has spread throughout the world. It has been so influential that the words yin and yang are now part of the vocabulary of Western languages.

Some of the typical characteristics of yin are mellow, yielding, unfathomable, discursive, and sensitive; those of yang are the opposites (Table 4.1).

Table 4.1   Yin and Yang Characteristics

Yang 阳	Yin 阴
Male	Female
Light	Darkness
External	Internal
Day	Night
Strong	Mellow
Rigid & Unyielding	Flexible & Yielding
Hard	Soft
Transparent	Unfathomable
Hot, Dry	Cool, Moist
Fast, Hurried	Slow, Patient
Analytical	Discursive
Insensitive	Sensitive

---

[7] For example, Chapter 6 of Hong (2016).

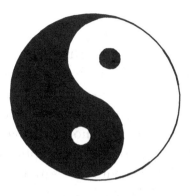

Fig. 4.1 Symbol of yin and yang

Applications of the Yin-Yang Principle in medicine

Several relationships make up the Yin-Yang Principle.

1. **Mutual opposition** (阴阳对立). One of the principles of yin and yang is that they oppose and restrain each other. If you observe the symbol of yin and yang in Fig. 4.1, you will notice that the dark portion representing yin exercises a restraining influence on the white portion representing yang. Likewise, yang has an opposing, controlling influence on yin.
2. **Interdependence of yin and yang** (阴阳互根). Although they restrain each other, yin and yang also depend on each other for their existence. Notice from the symbol of yin-yang that each wraps around and supports the other. One could not exist without the other.

   This seemingly paradoxical situation in which two forces oppose but are also dependent on each other is one of the deep insights derived from Daoist philosophy. Yet that is much the way the universe and life inside are structured. If there is light, there must be darkness to contrast, otherwise the notion of light would not exist. And, as Daoist sage Laozi opined in the Dao De Jing, "It is because everyone under Heaven recognizes beauty as beauty that the idea of ugliness exists."[8]

When we extend this idea to behaviour in human society, we understand better why Chinese philosophy emphasises balance in many ways. Somebody who opposes and restrains you is also somebody on whom you may be dependent. In a healthy democracy, there must be checks and balances. A ruling party that governs unfettered, with no opposing forces to keep it honest, eventually falls into power corruption and decadence.

In a corporate management organisation, you need analytical, transparent and forceful persons among its leaders, but you also benefit from the leavening influence of softer and flexible managers. These managers are more forgiving of human errors and make allowances for deviation from rigid rules that could cramp initiative and entrepreneurship to the detriment of the organisation.

In the historical rivalry between the civilisations of Athens and Sparta in ancient Greece, Sparta became overly yang in nature, run by leaders who revelled in power and emphasized military training. Soft yin skills were repressed. Sparta eventually perished.

3. **Yin and yang wax and wane** (阴阳消长). They rise and fall in cycles. There will be times that yang is dominant, then begins to decline as yin rises and becomes dominant. An obvious example is the day and night cycle. Day is yang and night is yin. When the sun rises at dawn, yang starts to assert itself over the receding yin of the night and early morning. By noon yang reaches a peak, then gradually declines and begins to give way to yin at dusk. Yin reaches a peak at midnight, and the cycle repeats.

This yin-yang cycle has implications for good living habits. We should rest and sleep in the yin phase of the cycle and be active and perform energetic tasks when yang is flourishing. We should not do demanding work at night but rather prepare for sleep

---

[8] See Hong (2020) p.48.

Yin and Yang Daily Cycle

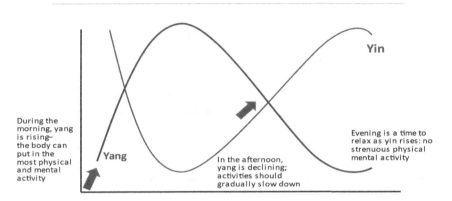

Fig. 4.2   The daily yin-yang cycle

early so that by midnight, when yin is at the peak, we are already soundly asleep and the body recuperates from the toils of the yang-dominated day. The best time for physical exercise is early in the morning when yang is rising rather than in the evening when rising yin beckons us to relax and rest.

The yin-yang cycle can be seen in the four seasons. After a cold winter, yin wanes as the weather begins to warm with the beginning of spring. In mid-summer, yang reaches a peak, then declines into autumn as yin waxes and yang wanes. Yin reaches a peak at winter solstice (冬至). Old man winter then begins to wane, only occasionally showing its recalcitrance with an early spring heavy snowfall. *Lichun* (立春) marks the beginning of spring as yang waxes again. And so the cycles continue interminably.

4. **Mutual transformation** (阴阳转化). When yang waxes to the extreme stage and becomes over-exuberant, it can turn into the opposite yin. Likewise extreme yin can turn into yang. A common example of this is summer solstice when summer yang heat peaks, yin begins to wax and take over and temperatures start to

fall. A more dramatic example is when a man suffers from a high temperature and his lungs are filled with internal heat, and his *zhengqi* (healthy qi) is exhausted. His face turns pale and limbs cold, and he shivers as yin takes over.

The mutual transformation of yin and yang would appear to be a somewhat abstruse subject and is not often applied to medical practice. However, the reader should take note that this aspect of yin yang relationship exists.

4.2 Medical Applications of the Yin-Yang Principle

Yin and yang characteristics are used extensively to describe substances and physiological conditions in Chinese medicine. For example, qi embodies energy and movement and is yang in character. In contrast, blood is yin, and runs deep and quietly nourishes the body. An overly warm body has a predominance of yang, and an overly cool body an excess of yin. The back of the body that is warmed by the sun is yang, while the more protected front is yin.

The Circadian cycle

We have observed earlier that the Yin-Yang Principle prescribes that we work by day and rest after dusk, and sleep before yin peaks at midnight. Modern medicine has made the same discovery and has been able to explain the profound physiological effects of the circadian cycle on the healthy functioning of the human body. The pineal gland located beneath the forehead can sense changes in light and instruct the body to be active or relax according to the time of the day. Three scientists won the 2017 Nobel prize in medicine/physiology for demonstrating the effects of the circadian cycle on the healthy functioning of the body. The Nobel citation declared, "With exquisite precision, our inner clock adapts our physiology to the dramatically different phases of the day. The clock regulates critical functions such as behaviour, hormone levels, sleep, body temperature and metabolism."[9] The scientists had indeed made an important contribution to medical science with their detailed studies of physiological biomarkers that change within the Circadian cycle. However, some TCM physicians feel that some acknowledgment could have been made of ancient Chinese wisdom in yin-yang daily cycles of life, which preceded by several millennia the prize-winning studies of their biomedical effects.

Yin-yang imbalances that cause illness

There are several kinds of yin-yang imbalance which cause the body to fall ill. Let's look at two common examples. Fig. 4.3 shows yin and yang in balance in a healthy body.

In example 1 (Fig. 4.4), yang is in excess. This could be due to a number of reasons. One possibility is eating too much "heaty" (warm) foods or tonics, hence causing the yang in our body to become unduly strong. This generates excess heat whilst yin stays at the normal level. This condition can express itself in the body feeling warm, a sore throat, red tongue and fast pulse. The person is said to have excess or sthenic heat (*shi re* 实热). Treatment is by dispelling the excess heat using heat-clearing herbs such as honeysuckle flower (金银花).

In example 2 (Fig. 4.5) which happens commonly in hot climates, yang is at a normal level, but yin has been damaged or weakened

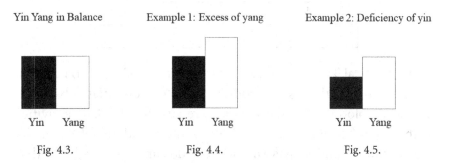

Yin Yang in Balance	Example 1: Excess of yang	Example 2: Deficiency of yin
Yin Yang	Yin Yang	Yin Yang
Fig. 4.3.	Fig. 4.4.	Fig. 4.5.

[9] Nobel Prize for Medicine or Physiology (2017).

from overworking, exposure to hot weather and excessive sweating. As a result, there is a deficiency of yin and consequently yang becomes relatively strong. In this situation, heat is also produced. This kind of heat is known as the deficiency heat or asthenic heat (*xu re* 虚热). Heat comes not from excessive yang but by default because yin has been weakened, making yang appear strong. The usual symptoms are dryness in the eyes and skin, thirst that is not quenched by drinking water, and a feeling of vexatiousness. Besides people who are subjected to heat, sweating and overwork, women in the menopausal stage also tend to have this condition. Such women would typically present symptoms such as hot flashes, night sweating and dry eyes and skin. The remedy is not to expel heat, but rather to nourish yin using herbs like wolfberry seed (枸杞子) and lily bulb (百合) that can help to strengthen yin.

4.3 The Viscera: *Zang* and *Fu*-organs

In TCM, there are five *zang* (脏) organs, each with a matching *fu* (腑) organ that functions closely with it. Hence the term "*zang fu*" refers to the viscera in the body.

Zang 脏 ("solid")	*Fu* 腑 ("hollow")
Liver 肝	Gall Bladder 胆
Heart 心	Small Intestine 小肠
Spleen 脾	Stomach 胃
Lung 肺	Large Intestine 大肠
Kidney 肾	Bladder 膀胱

By classical TCM theory, *zang* organs are considered to be solid. Their main function is to produce and store essential substances such as qi, blood and essence which are vital for the daily activities of the body. The *fu* organs are hollow and mostly involved in the transportation and transformation of substances in the body that flow through them. For example, the kidney stores essence which is necessary for the growth and development of the body besides processing urine, whereas the bladder stores urine that needs to be excreted from the body.

In addition to the five *fu*-organs, there is a notional *fu*-organ known as the "triple burner" or *sanjiao* (三焦) which consists of the hollow trunk of the body from the chest to the abdomen, containing all the *zang* and *fu* organs. The *sanjiao* is also known as the triple energizer as it energizes the transmission of qi and water up and down the trunk of the body.

Functions of the *zang-fu* organs

The heart and small intestine

The heart propels blood and participates in the production of blood to nourish the body. The heart also governs mental activities through the nourishing function of heart blood and heart yin. A person with deficiency in blood would often experience insomnia, poor memory, and difficulty in concentrating as there is insufficient blood to nourish the mind.

The small intestine receives chyme from the stomach. It separates nutrients from waste material and absorbs the nutrients and part of the water from the chyme.

The lung and large intestine

The lung governs respiratory qi as well as production and circulation of qi. Respiratory qi refers to the qi that we breathe in and out through our respiratory system. The lung also regulates the water passage for circulation and excretion purposes. The *Huangdi Neijing* makes the interesting observation that the lung is situated at the upper trunk of the triple burner, which is the highest point of the water passage and thus it can divert water to other parts of the body.

The large intestine receives food waste from the small intestine, absorbs part of the water in it, and transmits the waste downward in the form of stool for excretion.

The liver and gallbladder

The liver has the function of dredging and regulating, which means it helps to ensure the smooth passage of qi. Healthy qi flow is also needed for good blood flow, which helps to promote circulation of blood and metabolism, assists the stomach in digestion and regulates mental activity. The liver also stores blood and helps to regulate blood flow during menstruation.

The gallbladder is connected to the liver. It stores and secrets bile produced by the liver.

The spleen and stomach

The spleen governs transportation and transformation of food, absorbing nutrients and transforming them into qi and blood for the vital body activities. The spleen is known as the post-natal basis of life (后天之本) because it is the source of qi and blood made from nutrition. After birth, our bodies constantly require qi and blood to grow and function. When someone has spleen-qi deficiency, it means that the spleen is unable to absorb and transport the nutrients properly. As a result, they present symptoms such as poor appetite, lethargy, loose stools and abdominal bloating.

The stomach receives and digests food, transforming food to chyme to pass on to the small intestine. Stomach qi propels food downwards, hence the stomach is said to govern descent. Thus, dysfunction of the stomach can lead to bloating and diminished appetite.

Another function of the spleen is to "command" blood. This refers to its role in helping to retain blood within blood vessels, preventing it from leaking out and causing internal bleeding. Hence internal bleeding can sometimes be attributed to spleen qi deficiency.

The kidney and bladder

In TCM the kidney has the most complex functions, much beyond what is attributed to the kidney in Western medicine.

It is known as the prenatal base of life (先天之本) as it stores essence (*jing*), which governs growth, development, reproduction and ageing. Essence increases in a child as hair grows and teeth start to form. It rises further as puberty sets in, reaching a peak at the physical prime age of twenties and thirties, when the body is strongest and bountiful in energy. A child with a low level of essence from birth may experience slow growth, poor hair and teeth development, and develop a smaller build. For adults who have kidney deficiency, symptoms commonly appear in the reproductive system. Males may experience erectile dysfunction, and females a possible earlier onset of menopause.

Another function of the kidney is to govern water metabolism which includes the excretion of urine. In this narrow respect it is similar to the kidney in Western medicine.

As the kidney is located at the lower trunk of the body, it helps to receive qi that is inhaled from the lung. Only when kidney qi is adequate for receiving qi can the lung qi descend to the kidney. Weakness in this function can be seen in patients, particularly the elderly, who may experience shortness of breath and asthma.

The kidney also has warming and nourishing functions for internal organs. Kidney yang warms yang in all the organs, while kidney yin nourishes yin in the organs. Weakness in kidney yin in turn leads to deficiency in yin in the other *zang* organs.

The kidney also produces and nourishes marrow which in TCM includes not only bone marrow but also the spinal cord and brain marrow. Hence a person whose kidney essence is insufficient to produce marrow may suffer from dizziness, headache, and memory loss.

The bladder stores and discharges urine. Kidney qi is needed to transform water and turbid qi into urine, hence a misfunctioning of kidney qi leads to disorder in urine excretion.

4.4 The Five-Element Model

Besides yin yang, the other important TCM principle is *Wuxing* (五行), usually translated as the Five Elements, but also sometimes called the Five Phases. *Wuxing* has origins in ancient cosmology in which the world was made up of 5 elements: wood, water, fire, earth and metal. These were deemed to have interactive relationships with one another. [10]

One relationship is called inter-promotion. This uses the analogy of "mother promotes (generates) child". Wood promotes fire, fire promotes earth, earth promotes metal and metal promotes water, which in turn promotes wood (Fig. 4.6).

The other relationship is inter-restraint, by which the grandmother restrains the grandchild (Fig. 4.7).

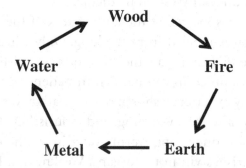

Fig. 4.6   The Five Elements

[10] Joseph Needham records some of the historical development of the five-element model in cosmology, pointing out that it had origins in and applications to relationship among the emperor and his ministers in ancient Chinese courts. See Needham (2016).

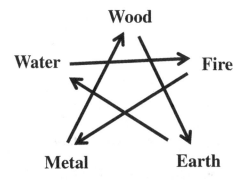

Fig. 4.7   Inter-restraint among the five elements

Applying the five-element model to the *zang* organs

TCM theory relates the properties of the five elements to the functions of the *zang* organs. For example, the kidney governs water metabolism, hence the kidney is assigned to the water element. The heart pumps blood that warms the body, hence it is assigned to the fire element. The spleen governs transportation and transformation of food into nutrients, just as the earth produces nutrients for the growth of the plants. Hence the spleen's functions match the properties of earth.

Application to therapy

Based on clinical experience, the ancients borrowed this model to put the five *zang* organs in the same cyclical combination (Fig. 4.8). This fitted their understanding of the relationships among these organs. Over time it was adopted as a guide for the diagnosis and treatment of disorders in these organs.

In inter-promotion, we tonify the mother to strengthen the child (虚者补其母). In other words, the health of the unborn child is dependent on the mother and the kind of nutrition she provides the child. This analogy is useful in TCM therapy. For example, in the treatment of cough with phlegm, most physicians would not only

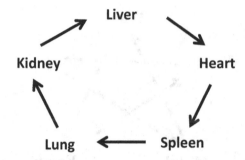

Fig. 4.8   Inter-promotion relationship among *zang* organs

treat the lung to clear the phlegm but also the spleen (its mother). Spleen tonics like *dangshen* (党参) are added in the prescription to strengthen spleen qi and *chenpi* (陈皮) to improve its flow. This strengthens the lung and prevents the production of phlegm. This is called tonifying the spleen to promote lung function.

Another example is the treatment of liver yin deficiency syndrome with symptoms such as dry eyes, vexatiousness, and internal heat. One method of therapy is to nourish the kidney (mother) to promote the liver (child) function, a technique known as "water nourishing wood" (滋水涵木). Hence, when physicians write prescriptions for this condition, herbs to nourish the kidney yin can be used in place of those that nourish the liver yin directly, or play a complementary role to those herbs.

The inter-restraint relationship may be applied to disorders in which one organ restrains another, as shown in Fig. 4.9.

Sometimes restraint is excessive, for example when the liver over-restrains the spleen. In these cases, it is necessary to inhibit the liver and strengthen the spleen (抑肝扶脾) to mitigate the effect of an over-exuberant liver.

Orthodox Chinese scholars regard the five-element model as some kind of immutable law of nature akin to the laws of physics. A more pragmatic view is to regard this as a model that closely captures the relationships among organs observed in their clinical

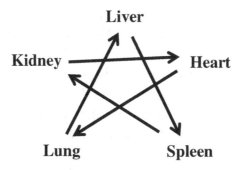

Fig. 4.9   Inter-restraint relationships among *zang* organs

work. In science, this is called a heuristic model, discovered through experimentation to be useful for explaining clinical findings. Hence the five-element model has become a useful heuristic tool for Chinese physicians in diagnosis and therapy.

4.5 Understanding the Nature of TCM Organs

In modern Western anatomy, the organs are defined as tissues that carry out specific functions. For example, the heart pumps blood throughout the body, the kidney filters blood to produce urine, and the stomach processes food to produce chyme that passes on to the small intestine for further digestion. They are also said to be "somatic structures", that is, they have defined shapes and locations in the body.

TCM organs may appear similar to organs in modern anatomy but are in actuality quite different. Modern TCM textbooks describe the *zang-fu* organs not as just somatic structures but as "syntheses of functional units" (综合性的功能单位), indicating that a number of diverse functions are incorporated in each organ.[11]

However, such a characterization of *zang-fu* organs is somewhat abstract if not also ambiguous. It also does not deal with the

---

[11] See, for example, Wu Changguo (2002).

anomaly that some of the organs have functions that are carried out, not in the location of the somatic structural unit, but in other places in the body. In fact, in the case of the spleen, the functions of digestion are carried out in the digestive tract and not at all in the somatic structure known as the spleen. The organ called the spleen in modern anatomy has nothing to do with digestion. It has instead an immune system function and also acts as a reservoir for blood.

What then is the best way to describe the TCM organ? We suggest that each organ should be regarded, not as a somatic structure, but as an entity that has a *cluster of functions*. There can be many functions within the cluster, as we have seen in the case of the kidney, which has at least five functions ranging from reproduction to warming the body organs.

Not being a somatic structure, the organ does not necessarily have one location. Take the spleen example again. It is involved in digestion, hence its functions include those attributed to the stomach, small and large intestines in modern anatomy, as well as the physiological mechanisms for the production of gastric and other digestive secretions. With modern knowledge of the microbiome system in the guts, we should probably also include gut flora as part of the spleen. The spleen in TCM also commands blood, keeping its flow within blood vessels. Hence the spleen should be described as a physiological unit with the functions of digestion and commanding blood. Its location within the body is no longer relevant, as it is not a somatic structure.

For historical reason, going back to ancient times when physicians thought that the somatic spleen governed digestion, we described it as a solid *zang* organ. In the light of our explanation of its functions, it would be more accurate to regard the spleen as the physiological representation of digestive and blood control functions.

One result of this approach is that we can now explain how, when a person has a diseased (somatic) spleen and has it surgically removed (splenectomy), the patient only needs an injection of certain vaccines to replace the spleen's immune system function. The patient's TCM spleen remains totally intact, and the digestive system works normally after the splenectomy!

Chapter 5

Causes, Diagnosis and Treatment of Illness

Why does one fall ill? Biomedicine (Western medicine) traces cause of disease to microbiological agents like viruses and bacteria, cellular disorders, malfunctioning of organs and declines in physiological systems like the cardiovascular and nervous systems.

Chinese medicine in ancient times did not know of the existence of microbiological agents. Nor did it understand the functioning of cells. Instead, it sought explanation for illness in external climatic factors and internal emotional factors.

To illustrate the difference in approaches of these two schools of medicine, consider the common cold. Biomedicine attributes the cold to the rhinovirus. But Chinese medicine attributes it to climatic stress like cold and wind. The cold pathogen can invade the body because of a decline in healthy qi due to lack of rest, not eating well, or emotional and physical stress. We know now that that a person with a cold has the rhinovirus in their nasal discharges. TCM would tend to view the condition of having a rhinovirus infection as the definition of the common cold. The rhinovirus is in the air, and anyone can catch it. But only those whose resistance (*zhengqi*) is weak and who have been exposed to weather would be infected by the virus. TCM finds it more useful to identify weak *zhengqi* and exposure to weather as the cause of the cold. Such an approach is useful because it shows the way to avoid or prevent colds.

In general, for infections due to an invading pathogen, TCM also explains that there are two ways by which the body reacts. If the body has enough *zhengqi* left, it is able to do battle with the invading pathogen. The body warms up and develops symptoms such as fever, a reddish complexion, and sweating. This is an example of an "excess" condition or excess syndrome (*shizheng* 实证). On the other hand, if *zhengqi* is in a poor state, the body may succumb and become weaker as the pathogen takes hold. This weakened condition is said to be a deficiency condition, or a deficiency syndrome or (*xuzheng* 虚证). Typical symptoms seen in a deficiency condition are lethargy, breathlessness, poor appetite, and a pale complexion.

Let us now look in more detail at climatic and emotional factors that cause illness.

5.1 External Climatic Factors as Causes of Illness

Climatic factors comprise six external pathogens (*liuyin* 六淫): wind, cold, summer heat, fire, dryness and dampness. These pathogenic factors are closely related to the weather and the seasons. Under natural conditions when the body is in harmony with the nature, these climatic factors do not attack and invade the body to cause illnesses. However, when there is a disruption in harmony, such as being inadequately clothed for the cold weather, and at the same time the body's internal defences are weak, these climatic factors would invade the body and cause illness.

Each climatic factor is more prevalent during a certain season. For example, spring tends to be windier, summer has heat and fire, late summer is damp, autumn is dry and winter is cold.

Wind tends to float, move and change. Illnesses caused by the wind pathogenic factor are characterized by sudden onset, fast progression and mobility. Mobility has the main symptoms of tremours, dizziness, and spasms. The site of attack of wind pathogens is usually the upper respiratory tract. Hence a common component cause of common colds is wind. For this reason, the common cold is also called *shangfeng* (伤风) or "damage by wind".

Summer heat tends to dry up fluids in the body. Typical symptoms of illnesses caused by summer heat pathogens include thirst, a flushed complexion, sweating, dry stools, high fever, and a fast pulse. Fire has similar characteristics to those of summer heat, the main difference being that the damage by fire is wider and deeper in the body.

Dampness has the characteristic of being heavy and sticky, with a tendency to move downward and attack the spleen. Owing to its sticky nature, dampness causes stagnation in qi and the body consequently develops abdominal bloatedness and chest discomfort. Other symptoms associated with dampness are sticky loose stools, lethargy, heavy limbs, and a poor appetite.

Dryness tends to attack the lung and dry up body fluids. This may explain why most people tend to get dry coughs with scanty sputum in the autumn season. Dryness is also associated with dry throat, mouth and nose, hard stools, and less urine.

Cold tends to contract, coagulate and destroy yang qi. Cold pathogens usually cause symptoms such as pain, aversion to cold and poor qi and blood flow.

5.2 Emotional and Internal Factors as Causes of Illness

Many illnesses are self-inflicted by poor management of our emotions. Unlike the climatic pathogens which are external (exogenous) factors, seven emotions are internal (endogenous) factors capable of causing damage to the internal organs.

In TCM, poor management of a particular emotion is deemed to affect the functions of a specific organ. Excessive indulgence in joy or sexual pleasure adversely affects the heart. Anger or a vile temper damages the liver. Too much continuous thinking, or contemplation, damages the spleen. Grief hurts the lung (and we sigh.) Fear injures the kidney, fright harms the heart, and anxiety the lung and liver.

Many of these emotions are captured in the popular but loose usage of the word "stress". Depending on the context in which stress is used, it could refer to any one of the above emotions, or a combination of them. The kind of stress that is long-term and unremitting is associated with contemplation and anxiety.

Contemplation damages the spleen, whilst anxiety and anger hurt the liver, which in turn passes it to the spleen and stomach. Hence in high-stress societies like those in Hong Kong, New York, Singapore and Tokyo, dysfunction of the spleen is particularly prevalent. This may lead to indigestion, irritable bowel syndrome and chronic fatigue.

Working long hours, excessive physical exertion, or overindulgence in sex strain the body and affect internal flows and balance. Overindulgence in sex also harms the kidneys and results in low kidney qi, which may age the body and affect its resistance to disease in the long run. On the other hand, too much idleness such as sitting on the couch all day results in poor qi and blood flows which in turn can evolve into a variety of troublesome conditions.

Other causes of illness are toxic chemicals and harmful organisms (insects and poisonous animals), improper diet, and phlegm and blood stasis. Improper diet such as strongly flavoured, cold or excessive food consumption can result in dampness and heat and cause stagnation of spleen qi with symptoms of abdominal bloatedness, loose stools, and poor appetite. Phlegm and blood stasis are pathogens internal to the body. We discuss them in the next section on syndromes.

5.3 TCM Syndromes

In chapter 3 we introduced the concept of the TCM syndrome (*zheng* 证) as central to TCM thinking on the nature of illness. Chinese medicine recognises syndromes as the most basic level of illness. Diagnosing and treating syndromes is the core of TCM.

TCM syndromes comprise basic syndromes as well as complex syndromes in which several syndromes are present together.

Basic syndromes

1. Cold and heat. Heat is identified by symptoms like aversion to heat, flushed complexion, thirst with preference for cold drinks,

restlessness/insomnia, yellowish sputum, brownish and scanty urine, dry stools, and a reddish tongue. The cause of this syndrome may be an excess of yang or deficiency of yin. The cold syndrome has symptoms of aversion to cold, no inclination to drink water, a pale complexion and light-coloured tongue, loose stools, frequent and higher volume urination.

2. Dryness and dampness. Dampness is accompanied by a feeling of heaviness in the head, chest discomfort, loss of appetite, lassitude, loose stool, and sticky fur on the tongue. Dryness is caused by insufficiency of body fluids with dryness of mouth, nose, throat and skin, scanty urine and dry stool. It tends to impair the lung, causing dry coughs with little phlegm.

3. Deficiency and Excess. Deficiency and excess can apply to qi, blood, yin and yang. The following are characteristics of deficiency and excess syndromes:

Deficiency syndrome 虚证	Excess syndrome 实证
• Deficiency of healthy qi • Body needs replenishment • Need for tonics and tonifying interventions (e.g. herbs, acupuncture)	• Adequate level of healthy qi • Exuberance of pathogenic factors • Need to dissipate pathogens

4. External and Internal. Syndromes can also be classified as external or internal.

External syndrome 表证	Internal syndrome 里证
Early stages of illness; invasion by external/infectious pathogens	Affects the organs, qi and blood etc.; chronic diseases
Acute fever, aversion to cold/wind, headache, sneeze, blocked nose, runny nose, sore throat, mild cough, floating pulse	All other diseases besides external syndrome

Complex syndromes

A complex syndrome can combine several basic syndromes. It can also be specific to a body location. For example, a patient may have the dampness syndrome at the same time as the heat syndrome. He is then regarded as having the heat dampness syndrome, which requires therapy to remove dampness and dispel heat. Just by removing the dampness alone, or heat alone, will not resolve the syndrome.

A further complexity arises when heat dampness is specifically located in particular organs, for example heat dampness syndrome of the stomach and spleen. This then requires treatment with herbs that are effective for removing heat and dampness in the spleen and stomach.

Other examples of complex syndromes are yin deficiency of the kidney and qi stagnation of the liver with internal heat.

During the progression of an illness, syndromes are in a dynamic state and will change over time. This explains why it is not advisable to take the same prescription for a long period of time without consulting a physician as to whether the underlying syndrome of the illness has changed.

Phlegm 痰

Phlegm in TCM usage is much wider in meaning than the sticky phlegm one coughs out from the throat. It is a syndrome that begins with dampness which left untreated progresses to a less viscous fluid called "rheum" (*yin* 饮), and finally to viscous phlegm. Phlegm in the broad sense covers both thin rheum and sticky viscous phlegm. Sticky phlegm is seen as thick mucus that accompanies cough and sneezing. Rheum is insidious and without form, and can be challenging to eliminate. Phlegm and rheum hinder the flow of blood and qi. They can cause confusion of mind, chest oppression, numbness in limbs, edema, convulsions and conditions leading to strokes. From ancient times, Chinese medicine has blamed phlegm for many diseases of unknown cause, hence the expression "Strange diseases are caused by phlegm" (百病多由痰作祟).

Blood stasis 血瘀

Blood stasis is a syndrome that results from stagnation of blood and disturbance in circulation. The underlying pathology most of the time is qi deficiency, hence we could say that qi deficiency is the root and blood stasis is the resulting syndrome. Blood stasis hinders flows and physiological processes. The syndrome is usually manifested as stabbing pain, dark (purple) coloured tongue and a thin, taut pulse. In TCM theory, it is one of the underlying conditions encouraging the development of coronary heart disease.

We shall come across blood stasis often when we study chronic illnesses. Blood stasis is common among patients who have suffered long illness, or who have received severe treatments like chemotherapy and radiation therapy. It tends also to occur more frequently among the elderly.

5.4 TCM Diagnosis

TCM diagnosis differs from Western medical diagnosis in relying purely on human observation (visual, tactile, smell, sounds) and the patient's detailed description of their own condition. Through these observations, the physician makes inferences regarding the particular syndrome(s) that trouble the patient. Once the syndrome is identified, the physician applies therapeutic principles to formulate a prescription to address the syndrome. *Bianzheng lunzhi* (辩证论治), or identifying the syndrome and treating accordingly, is the essence of Chinese diagnosis and therapy. It addresses the illness at its root and treats the underlying cause.

The Four Examinations 四诊

The method of TCM diagnosis comprises four procedures: inspection (望), smells and sounds (闻), questions (问) and pulsation (切).

Inspection

To inspect means to examine the physical appearance of the patient. This includes looking at the whole body and specific parts of it, particularly the tongue. When we are looking at the whole body, we are trying to obtain general information by examining the patient's skin complexion, behaviour, and posture. Importantly the physician notes spirit of the eyes (*yanshen* 眼神), whether they indicate good reserves of energy and look well or tired.

Inspecting the tongue is an essential diagnostic tool in Chinese medicine. The colour, shape and flexibility of the tongue reflect the conditions of the organs, qi, and blood. The fur of the tongue is the layer of coating on the tongue which cannot be removed, except temporarily, by scraping the tongue. It indicates the nature of the pathogenic factors in the body and their interaction with the healthy qi of the patient. For example, a red-coloured tongue indicates that there is heat in the body. A pale tongue reflects a deficiency in qi, blood or yang. A red tongue with greasy yellow fur points to heat-dampness syndrome.

The normal tongue of a healthy person should be light reddish in colour with thin white fur. Deviations in the appearance of the tongue and fur from normal are rich in information, helping the physician to determine the underlying syndrome(s) of the patient.

Smells and sounds

These refer to olfaction and listening. The examining physician may be able to detect odours of the body, breath, sputum, mucus, and even the sweat of the patient. The physician listens to the patient's voice and speech, looking for signs of cough, unusual breathing, hiccups or belching. A patient who is coughing loudly with foul sourish stench from the sputum usually has heat phlegm excess syndrome. But when a patient coughs very gently, speaks softly with effort and shows breathlessness, it is likely there is a deficiency syndrome.

Questioning

To ascertain the occurrence, development and treatment of the illness, the physician inquires into the patient's medical and family history, chief complaint, history of the present illness and presenting symptoms such as diet, sleep, urination and bowel habits.

Pulse-taking and palpation

Taking the pulse by placing three fingers over the wrist of the patient helps to reveal more information on the inner conditions of the body (Fig 5.1).

Taking pulse is not just feeling its rate but also its texture and depth. There are altogether 28 pathological pulses in TCM. Each pulse has its own specific feel and characteristics relating to one or

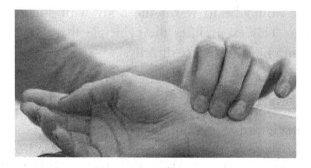

Fig 5.1   Pulse-taking

Table 5.1   Varieties of Pulse

Pulse	Description	Clinical significance
Floating 浮	Can be felt under light pressure, becomes slightly weak with more pressure	1. External syndrome 2. Internal syndrome due to severe deficiency of blood/essence
Sunken 沉	Can only be felt under heavier pressure	Internal syndrome
Slippery 滑	Smooth like rolling of beads on an abacus	1. Phlegm syndrome 2. Retention of food 3. Deficiency heat syndrome 4. Normal pulse in pregnancy
Thin or thready 细	Can be felt under light pressure. Weak and thin as a thread	1. Qi and blood deficiency 2. Dampness syndrome
Taut 弦	Feels like the string of a violin	1.Liver and gall bladder disorders 2. Pain 3. Retention of phlegm and fluid

more syndromes. Some of the common pulses encountered in clinical practice are shown in Table 5.1.

The strength of TCM diagnosis is that it is patient centric. The treatment regimen is tailored to the patient rather than the disease itself. Two persons may come in with a cold but, based on their presenting symptoms, one may be diagnosed with a heat syndrome whereas the other a cold syndrome. The therapy for the heat syndrome would be to dispel the heat whereas that for the cold syndrome it would be to warm the body with suitable medical interventions. This exemplifies the principle that TCM treats the syndromes and not the disease directly.

Syndrome Differentiation

After gathering information from the four examinations, the physician identifies the pattern, that is, differentiates the syndrome. There are several systems of classification of syndromes in TCM diagnosis. We describe here two main ones often used together in clinical practice.

The eight-principle method of diagnosis (八纲辩证)

The eight principles are yin yang, external versus internal, cold versus heat, and deficiency versus excess (asthenia versus sthenia).

The external and internal characterizations are used to differentiate the location and stages of the illness, whether they are at the surface/skin level of the body (external syndrome) or deeper down to the levels of qi, blood and the vital organs (internal syndrome). Generally, external syndromes are at an early stage and are easier to treat. Internal syndromes take a longer time as they involve the impairment of qi, blood, body fluids, and possibly the vital organs.

The cold and heat principles are used to differentiate the nature of the illness that reflect the level of yin and yang in the body. A heat syndrome is due to an excess of yang or deficiency of yin. A cold syndrome is due to an excess of yin or deficiency of yang.

The deficiency and excess principles reflect the state of the healthy qi (*zhengqi*) and pathogenic factors. A deficiency syndrome indicates a weakness in the *zhengqi* causing the body to be unable to fight off the pathogens. To address this syndrome, the body will need replenishment with tonics. The excess syndrome is due to an exuberance of pathogenic factors in the presence of adequate healthy qi, and the body is thus putting up a fight.

Differentiation by qi, blood and body fluids

Syndromes can also be differentiated by disorders of qi, blood or body fluids. Examples of disorders of qi are qi stagnation and qi deficiency and, for blood disorders, blood stasis, blood deficiency, and blood-heat syndromes. Body fluids disorders include fluid deficiency and the phlegm syndrome.

In a typical diagnosis, the physician may identify syndromes from the different classifications and apply them to a particular patient. For example, a patient may be diagnosed as having heat dampness with qi deficiency.

5.5 Therapeutic Principles

After a syndrome is differentiated, we can apply the appropriate therapy to treat the syndromes. The principle involved is to treat a given condition with an opposing balancing effect:

- Tonify if there is deficiency
- Purge if there is excess
- Cool if there is heat
- Warm if there is cold
- Dry if there is dampness
- Moisten if there is dryness
- Regulate or promote the flow if there is stagnation of qi
- Promote blood flow if there is stagnation (stasis) of blood
- Expel if there is wind
- Resolve it if there is phlegm

The mode of therapy chosen by the physician can be in the form of herbs, acupuncture, moxibustion or tuina, or a combination of either one of these modalities.

It has often been observed that a patient who sees two different physicians can be diagnosed with the same syndromes yet receive different treatments. This may happen because there may be slight differences in judgment and emphasis involved in the choice of therapy. For example, one physician may place more emphasis on making the patient comfortable more quickly by focussing treatment of the syndrome that troubles the patient the most, which could be heat. Another physician may prescribe a formulation that is strong in removing dampness as the heat is relatively mild, but the dampness is felt to be more serious long term in damaging the patient's health.

Chapter 6

The Nature and Properties of Herbs

Traditionally, when we think about Chinese medicinal herbs, we tend to conjure up the image of a bitter concoction boiled in a clay pot. Although most Chinese herbs are prepared this way for consumption as medicine, many herbs such as Chinese yam, *danngui* (angelica root) and lily bulb are regularly used as food ingredients in family meals. Such herbs are favoured for cooking as they have more pleasant taste and can serve both as medicine as well as food.

The wonder of nature is that the humble root of a plant, or its leaves, bark, flowers and seeds, all have potential medicinal value. Most of these plant parts have been carefully studied over thousands of years for their health and therapeutic effects by generations of herbalists and physicians.

The accumulated experience with these herbs has been recorded in various volumes of Chinese pharmacopeia. The earliest extant manual on herbs was the work of legendary herbalist Shen Nong. It contained detailed descriptions of 365 herbs that he personally tested for toxicity and side effects. The most comprehensive record of Chinese herbs to date, first published in 1578 during the Ming dynasty, is the *Compendium of Materia Medica* (*Bencao Gangmu* 本草纲目). This classic has since served as a reference text by Chinese physicians and pharmacists. It covers 1892 items, inclusive of medicines of animal and mineral origins. An encyclopaedic and scholarly work based on meticulous studies and experimentation, it is lasting testimony to the empirical scientific tradition of Chinese medicine. From ancient times, TCM has relied on clinical evidence provided by detailed observation, record and analysis.

In modern times, most Chinese herbs have been analysed in the laboratory and in clinical trials for therapeutic properties, toxicity, and side effects. Knowledge and experience from these studies by generations of physicians have been carefully documented in modern texts. Much work remains to be done as the variety of herbs is enormous and their biochemical complexity is of a much higher order than that of modern pharmaceuticals. Just a single herb typically contains dozens and sometimes over a hundred different ingredients and molecules, in contrast to a Western drug that usually comprises a single chemical known as its active ingredient.

Plant sources of herbs include roots, grasses, leaves, barks, stems, flowers, seeds and fruits. For example, ginseng is a root; chrysanthemum is a flower; peppermint is a leaf; wolfberries are fruits and *duzhong* (杜仲) is the bark of a tree. Medicines can also be derived from minerals and animals. Mineral sources include oyster shells, magnetite and haematite. Even creatures like scorpions, centipedes and parts of animals such as the tortoise shell are usable as medicine.

For ease of reference, all medicinal ingredients used in TCM will be termed "herbs" in this book.

6.1 Properties and Flavours of Herbs

There are many ways by which we can classify herbs. They can be classified according to their therapeutic actions, that is, in what ways they can be used for healing. This is a large subject and will be covered in detail in chapters 8 to 11 of this book. You will discover that each herb has more than one therapeutic action even though in textbooks they are organised according to their main action.

At a more basic level, we can classify herbs according to their properties and flavours.

Properties of Herbs

The property of a herb refers to its nature, whether it has a warming or cooling effect on the body. Hence, herbs are classified according to whether they are hot, warm, neutral, cool or cold. Excluding the neutral property, these are also known as "the four natures" or *siqi* (四气).

The property of a herb indicates its effect on pathogenic heat and cold. Herbs that are warm in nature, such as Chinese cinnamon, have a warming effect on the body and are used to treat cold syndromes. Herbs with cool property, such as chrysanthemum flower, are used to treat heat syndromes. Herbs that are hot have stronger effects than warm herbs and are used to treat more severe cold syndromes such as kidney yang deficiency. Being warmer in nature, if used inappropriately they can have troublesome side effects of internal heat with symptoms such as constipation and a sore throat. Dried ginger is an example of a hot herb.

Herbs that are cold in nature have stronger cooling actions than those that are classified as cool. Hence, they are used to treat severe heat syndromes such as exuberance of stomach fire. Inappropriate or excess usage of cold herbs over a prolonged period can impair spleen yang with symptoms such as loose stools, aversion to cold, and poor appetite. A common herb with cold property is gypsum (*shigao* 石膏).

Herbs that are neutral in nature can be used in both heat and cold syndromes. The therapeutic actions for this group of herbs are generally milder and do not have many contraindications. As they are well tolerated by people with different constitutions, they are suitable for use as food. Examples of neutral herbs are Chinese yam and lotus seeds (莲子 *lianzi*).

Flavours of herbs

The flavour of a herb is akin to its taste. However in some instances it may not have quite the taste that we expect. For example, liquorice

Table 6.1　Flavours of Herbs

Flavours	Actions	Examples
Pungent 辛	Dispersion 解表	*Bohe* (Peppermint) 薄荷
Sweet 甘	Tonifies 补 Moisturises 润 Harmonizes 和	*Gancao* (Liquorice) 甘草
Sour 酸	Arresting 收敛固涩	*Wuweizi* 五味子
Bitter 苦	Clearing heat 泻火	*Xiakucao* 夏枯草
Salty 咸	Softens 软坚	*Mangxiao* 芒硝

(*gancao* 甘草) has a sweet flavour in TCM terminology but may not actually taste sweet the way that sugar is sweet.

The five flavours (五味) are pungent (辛), sweet (甘), bitter (苦), sour (酸), and salty (咸) (Table 6.1).

Herbs that are pungent have the actions of dispersing and promoting qi and blood flow. In TCM, to disperse is to dispel the pathogens from the body surface, usually by sweating. Most herbs that are used to treat exogenous (external) syndromes are pungent. Examples are ginger and peppermint leaf.

Herbs that are sweet have the actions of nourishing, moistening, and harmonising. This is seen in most tonics, used to treat deficiency in qi, blood, yin or yang. Wolfberries and red dates are examples of tonics that are sweet.

The effects of bitter herbs are heat clearing and drying, which means that they can be used to treat heat syndromes. Expelling or purging the heat or fire from the body is through urination or defecation. Examples of heat-clearing herbs are *xiakucao* (夏枯草), used to purge liver fire, and *dahuang* (大黄) for expelling heat via defecation.

Herbs that are sour are said to have an arresting action, which means that they can treat profuse sweating, diarrhoea, frequent urination, and excessive vaginal white discharge (leucorrhoea 带下) or seminal fluids. One example is *wuweizi* (五味子).

Lastly, a herb that is salty can soften hard nodules and masses and promote defecation. One example is *mangxiao* (芒硝).

Many herbs have combinations of flavours. For example, *danggui* (当归), a warm blood tonic, is both sweet and pungent, so it can nourish blood as well as promote blood flow. Hence, it is used in formulations for regulating menstrual disorders caused by blood deficiency with blood stasis.

Besides property and flavour, another characteristic of a herb is its preferential effect on particular organs. This is known as *meridian tropism*. As we shall see in chapter 12, the human body has meridians along which qi flows. The main meridians notionally end in organs; hence the term meridian tropism describes the routes along which the herb's action flows to reach the preferred organs. For example, the yin tonic wolfberry is associated with the liver and kidney meridians, hence its use in formulations for treating liver and kidney yin deficiencies.

Most herbs in TCM have more than one flavour each, and more than one preferred meridian. However, each herb can only have one nature, which is used to guide its application for either a heat or a cold syndrome.

6.2 Toxicity

What does it mean for a herb to be toxic? This is important to understand because this term is sometimes abused and misunderstood.

"Toxic" in Western medicine means having a poisonous effect. It impairs the body tissues. The term is usually reserved for substances like arsenic that are harmful in small amounts. In other words, toxic substances like arsenic and mercury if taken in even small or moderate quantity can cause bad reactions, illnesses or even death.

However, in Chinese medicine, the word toxic or *du* (毒) has a wider usage. Only one of these usages corresponds to its meaning in Western medicine. Examples of its other meanings are as follows.

(a) It has special use for fighting certain pathogens, e.g., scorpions for endogenous (internal) wind pathogens. In this case, this toxicity is directed at the pathogens. Of course, when it kills the pathogens, it may have harmful side effects on the body and should be used with caution. There are popular sayings: "Use poison to fight poison (以毒攻毒)," and "Attack pathogens with poisonous herbs (毒药攻邪)." It means that something you must take may be directed to a pathogen even though it may have side effects on the body.

(b) Toxicity could mean having an undesirable side effect. For example, *shexiang* (麝香) (musk), used for resuscitation and promoting blood circulation to remove masses, can induce abortion. It must therefore be used in just the right amount to provide the desired therapeutic effect.

(c) Excessive use of a herb is harmful. For example, apricot kernel *(ku xingren* 苦杏仁*)*, used for relieving cough, has traces of cyanide. In practice, the bitter apricot kernel prescribed below a dosage limit is safe as the toxicity is minimal.

Generally, Chinese medicinal herbs are safe to consume if they are collected from the right sources and used in correct dosages. In fact, most of the herbs that are found in Chinese medical halls are processed. Processing can lower the level of toxicity of boiled herbs to a safe level for consumption.

6.3 Processing of Herbs

One can hardly find fresh or raw herbs in medical halls nowadays as herbs would normally have gone through some forms of processing before they are offered for retail sales. There are many types of processing. These include baking, stir-frying, washing, burning, calcination, simmering, and steaming. The purposes of processing herbs are:

(a) Removing or reducing toxicity. For example, *fuzi* (附子) for warming kidney yang needs to be boiled separately for at least 1 hour before mixing with other herbs.

(b) Promoting or enhancing therapeutic effect. When safflower (*honghua* 红花) is soaked in wine, it has a stronger effect of promoting blood flow.

(c) Modifying nature and actions. *Shengdihuang* (生地黄) or raw rehmannia is cool and used for clearing heat and cooling blood. After cooking in wine, it becomes *shudihuang* (熟地黄) or processed rehmannia, which has a warmer nature suitable for use as a tonic for nourishing blood.

(d) Facilitating decocting and ingestion of medicine, preparation, and storage of herbs. Cutting into smaller pieces and drying via sunning or baking help to prolong the storage life of the herbs while maintaining their properties. Silkworms (*jiangcan* 僵蚕) are usually stir-fried in salt to extend their shelf lives. Mineral herbs like oyster shells undergo burning, soaking in vinegar and crushing for easy dispensing. More importantly, this allows easier extraction of the active ingredients when brewed with other herbs in the formulation.

(e) Removing impurity and unpleasant tastes.

6.4 Compatibility of Herbs and Contraindications

A TCM formulation usually comprises several herbs. It is important to know how to combine the herbs effectively to increase the efficacy of therapy. How they are combined depends partly on the compatibility of the herbs with one another.

Compatibility

(a) Mutual reinforcement (*xiangxu* 相须). The herbs are compatible with each other and when put together, reinforce each other's therapeutic action. Herbs which are in this relationship usually have similar properties and actions. For example, safflower and peach seed (*taoren* 桃仁) are both blood flow promoting herbs. They are usually used together to mutually reinforce actions of enhancing blood flow and removing blood stasis.

(b) (Mutual) assistance (*xiangshi* 相使). This applies to herbs that do not have similar properties or main therapeutic actions. One herb would be the principal herb for therapeutic action while the other herb assists. For example, *huangqi* (黄芪) is a qi tonic used to replenish spleen qi. *Fuling* (茯苓), is the assisting herb with a diuretic as well as mild qi-tonifying action. It is used to enhance *huangqi*'s action for reducing water retention arising from spleen qi deficiency syndrome.

(c) Mutual restraint/detoxification (*xiangwei/xiangsha* 相畏/相杀). One herb reduces or removes the undesirable side effects such as toxicity in the other herb. For example, raw ginger (*shengjiang* 生姜) reduces the toxicity of *banxia* (半夏).

(d) Mutual inhibition (*xiange* 相恶). In this relationship, the combination of the herbs produces an undesirable effect of one reducing the effectiveness of the other. For example, the therapeutic actions of ginseng (人参) are weakened by radish (*laifuzi* 莱菔子), hence these two herbs should not be used together in a prescription.

(e) Incompatibility (*xiangfan* 相反) is a combination of two herbs that results in toxicity. There are a total of such 18 cases of incompatibility recorded in the Chinese pharmacopeia. One such pair is *wutou* (乌头) and *beimu* (贝母).

Contraindications

As in Western medicine, there can be contraindications between two herbs. This means that the herbs should be taken with caution and under medical supervision.

(a) During pregnancy, toxic herbs and herbs for promoting blood flow and removing blood stasis should be used with caution. This is because the enhanced blood flow may be too strong for the uterus, resulting in risk of miscarriage. Examples of such herbs are *shexiang, honghua, dahuang* (大黃) and *fuzi*.

(b) People with weak digestive systems are more sensitive to herbs that are of cool or cold in nature as these herbs tend to impair spleen and stomach functions by damaging yang, resulting in poor appetite, loose stools, and stomach discomfort. Examples of such herbs are *xiakucao* (夏枯草), *dahuang*, and gypsum.

(c) It is advisable not to take tonics when one is having a fever caused by external wind-heat or wind-cold pathogens. Tonics are mostly warm or hot in nature and taking them during fever may exacerbate the condition. The Chinese expression "闭门留寇," which means "close the door and trap the intruder," suggests that tonics trap the intruding pathogen inside the body. Likewise, taking tonics when having a cold is akin to providing the invading pathogens with nourishment.

6.5 Dosage

The dosage of herbs to be taken by patient is often decided by the physician based on the patient's condition, constitution, and medical history. This explains why it is always safer to consult a physician before taking medications. For example, more heat-clearing herbs should be given to someone who has a warm body constitution or suffers from a heat syndrome, compared to someone who has a cold body constitution or weak digestive system. In the latter case, the dosage of heat-clearing herbs should be lower and be prescribed for a shorter period.

In general, it is advisable for tonics to be taken before meals for better absorption of the nutrients. Herbs that may upset the stomach should be taken after meals, and calmatives before sleep.

6.6 Preparing Decoctions

Depending on the type of herbs, different herbs may require different methods of preparation.

Herbs that are toxic and in mineral form require boiling before cooking with other herbs. For example, *fuzi* needs to be boiled for one to one and a half hours to remove the toxins. Oyster shells need to be crushed and cooked for 20 to 30 minutes to fully extract the active ingredients.

Herbs such as peppermint that contain volatile components should be boiled only in the last five or ten minutes so that the heat will not disperse its volatile components and reduce their therapeutic actions. Herbs that are hairy or come in very fine particles or powdery form need to be isolated in sachets from the other herbs as remnants floating in the decoction may irritate the throat. Examples are *cheqianzi* (车前子) and *xuanfuhua* (旋覆花).

Chapter 7

Therapeutic Formulations

Traditionally, when people visit TCM physicians, they would leave with several bags of dried herbs to bring home to brew. Each bag of dried herbs contains the ingredients of medical formulation prescribed by the TCM physician. This practice carries on today in China and most countries around the world where TCM services are available. However, in recent years there has been increasing use of powdered extracts from herbs in place of raw herbs as extracts do not require boiling. These are kept in sachets that are convenient for storage and travelling.

The term for medical prescription or formulation is *fangji* (方剂). The word *fang* (方) means "method" and *ji* (剂) denotes a medical preparation. Hence *fangji* refers to a therapeutic formulation that is prescribed using a good or well-tried method, that is, a well-formulated medical prescription.

Chinese physicians discovered in ancient times that herbs can be combined in clever ways to achieve desired therapeutic results. This is somewhat like mixing a cocktail drink with an innovative combination of ingredients to yield a desired taste, or a food recipe to make an appetizing and nutritious dish. Unlike Western medicine, Chinese prescriptions are customized for the individual, taking into account the type and severity of the patient's syndromes as well as their constitution and state of health.

Hundreds of standard formulations were developed over thousands of years by Chinese physicians and most of them are still in use. In clinical practice, these formulations are usually modified by the physician to suit the patient's unique condition.

These standard formulations are classified according to their therapeutic effects. Because each formulation typically contains several herbs as a better result can usually be obtained from a cocktail of herbs than by using just one herb. This contrasts with the standard Western drug that contains one active chemical ingredient, with other ingredients only providing a base for the delivery of the active ingredient.

In Western medicine, a patient with several conditions, such as high blood pressure and diabetes, needs a number of different prescribed drugs, one for each condition. In the Chinese approach, one customized formulation is used to treat one or more illnesses presented as syndromes.

7.1 Forms of Prescriptions

Chinese medicine prescriptions come in many forms, the most common form being the decoction in which the herbs are boiled for an hour or longer to extract the useful ingredients.

Preparing a decoction

Ideally the decoction should follow the traditional procedure of boiling twice.

1. Soak the herbs in water for 20 minutes. There should be enough water to cover all the herbs.
2. Bring the herbs to boil and continue cooking with low heat for another 20 to 45 minutes, then decant into a big bowl.
3. Add water again to the pot of herbs and bring it to boil, then use low heat for another 30 minutes. Decant into the same bowl, thereby combining the product of the first and second boils to get a mixture of even concentration.
4. Divide the decoction into two separate bowls. One bowl can be consumed and the other covered and kept in the refrigerator for later use. Always drink the decoction warm.

Other forms of prescriptions

Other forms of prescriptions or formulations include powder, pill, honeyed boluses, concentrated pills, special pills, and medicated wine.

Honeyed boluses are much bigger than pills/concentrated pills and special pills. They have to be bitten and chewed before swallowing. These two forms of prescriptions are usually given for chronic illnesses and taken over a longer period.

Medicated wine is prepared from herbs soaked in strong wine with alcohol content in the range of 20% to 50%. Examples of such wines are the white *gaoliang* (高粱), rice wine and yellow wine. Liquor extractions are better for promoting blood circulation, moving qi along meridians, and expelling wind. Such wines should be taken in smaller amounts because of their alcohol concentration and strong therapeutic effects.

In modern times, with better processing technology and consumer demand for more convenient ways to take their medications, the forms of prescription commonly used in TCM clinics are powders, liquids or capsules/tablets that have been prepared by extraction techniques and presented in hygienic packaging.

7.2 The Principle of Combining Herbs

The general principle for combining herbs is analogous to a team effort, each herb playing one or two roles for the best overall therapeutic effect. These roles have colourful titles that are related to hierarchies in Chinese imperial courts. They are known as the monarch (*jun* 君), ministerial (*chen* 臣), adjuvant (*zuo* 佐), and guiding (*shi* 使) roles.

1. The Monarch herb plays the core therapeutic role as it targets the main syndrome. It is usually of higher dosage in the formulation.
2. The Ministerial herb assists the monarch herb by enhancing the monarch's therapeutic effect.

3. The Adjuvant herb plays a complementary role, supporting the monarch or/and minister herb by working on a related condition in the patient, or reducing toxicities and side effects, if any, of the monarch and ministerial herbs.

4. The Guiding herb helps direct the other herbs to the particular organs and harmonizes the overall therapeutic effect of the herbs in the formulation.

It is not necessary for every formulation to embody all four roles, although almost all formulations would have at least two to three of these roles covered by the constituent herbs. Of course, the simplest formulation of all is the single herb. For example, the ginseng decoction *dushentang* (独参汤), which contains only ginseng, plays the monarch role by invigorating qi in the body. This formulation is sometimes used to treat life-threatening conditions in which the person is critically ill and very weak. The dosage of ginseng used in these cases is relatively high.

It is not always the case that only one herb plays each role. Sometimes several herbs play the same role, each in its own way because of its particular flavour and properties that the formulation wants to utilize. We shall see examples of these when we examine some classical formulations.

We cover only a few classical formulations below. More formulations and their clinical applications are summarized in Annex 2 of the book.

7.3 Standard Formulations

There are hundreds of standard formulations commonly used by physicians. Some are classics that have stood the test of time. We begin with three of them, using them to illustrate the principles of combining herbs in the most optimal way.

Decoction of the Four Noble Herbs (*Sijunzi Tang* 四君子汤)

This is the foundation formulation for the qi deficiency syndrome. Its main therapeutic action is to tonify spleen qi, which is the main *zang* organ that produces qi. This decoction comprises four herbs: ginseng (人参) as the monarch herb, *baizhu* (白术) as the minister herb, poria (*fuling* 茯苓) as the adjuvant herb and honey-baked liquorice root (*zhigancao* 炙甘草), as the guiding herb. Ginseng is a qi tonic, and it targets the main syndrome of qi deficiency. *Baizhu* enhances the action of replenishing qi and removes dampness which often results from qi weakness of the spleen and stomach. *Fuling* eliminates dampness and strengthens the spleen. *Zhigancao*, a mild spleen qi tonic, completes the picture by harmonising the actions of the other herbs.

Extensions: This formulation can be extended for the same family of ailments but with different therapeutic emphasis. For example, adding *chenpi* (陈皮) and *banxia* (半夏) to the formulation creates the Decoction of the Six Noble Herbs (*Liujunzi Tang* 六君子汤) which addresses spleen deficiency with dampness and phlegm, characterized by poor appetite, loose stools, nausea, wet phlegm and thick or greasy white fur of the tongue.

When dampness and phlegm affect the flow of qi in the spleen in the patient, manifested in abdominal distension with frequent flatulence, qi-regulating herbs such as *muxiang* (木香) and *sharen* (砂仁) can be added to the Decoction of the Six Noble Herbs to regulate qi stagnation and restore qi flow in the spleen. This yields yet another formulation known as the *Xiangsha Liujunzi Tang* (香砂六君子汤).

Decoction of Four Ingredients (*Siwu Tang* 四物汤)

This is the basic formulation for tonifying blood, used to treat blood deficiency syndrome with symptoms of paleness of skin, eyelids and nails, insomnia, difficulty in concentration, dizziness, and pale white tongue with weak thready pulse.

In this decoction *shuidihuang* (熟地黄), the monarch herb, enriches blood and nourishes yin. *Danggui* (当归), the minister herb, enriches blood and strengthens the liver. *Chuanxiong* (川芎) and *baishao* (白芍) together play the adjuvant role. *Chuanxiong* promotes circulation of blood and qi. *Baishao* nourishes blood and the liver. There is no guiding herb. *Shudihuang, danggui* and *baishao* are all blood tonics for nourishing blood. Most blood tonics tend to impede the flow of qi, which in turn affects blood flow. Hence, the significance of adding *chuanxiong* in this formulation is to prevent blood stasis. The combination of the four herbs can enrich blood as well as regulate blood flow, thus providing a holistic therapeutic result.

Extensions: When blood deficiency is accompanied by blood stasis, the symptoms presented include stabbing pain and a pale tongue with dark spots. In this case, two blood flow promoting herbs *taoren* (桃仁) and *honghua* (红花) are added to create the formulation *Taohong Siwu Tang* (桃红四物汤). This has a stronger effect of promoting blood flow and removing stasis. This formulation is often used for irregular menstruation with blood clots.

Combining the Decoction of the Four Noble Herbs and the Decoction of the Four Ingredients gives us the popular formulation Decoction of Eight Precious Ingredients (*Bazhen Tang* 八珍汤). This formulation is much loved by housewives who buy them from medical halls and grocery stores for their daughters who have just completed menstruation. The decoction does indeed address both qi and blood deficiency syndromes in post-menstruation women. However, the formulation should be used in moderation, preferably with medical advice, as it is warm in nature with strong tonic properties and may not suit all constitutions. The monarch herbs are ginseng and *shudihuang*, with the principal effect of nourishing qi and blood. *Bazhen Tang* is normally used for prolonged weakness of qi and blood caused by excessive hemorrhage and depletion of qi.

Pill of Six Ingredients with Rehmannia (*Liuwei Dihuang Wan* 六味地黄丸)

This is a classic formulation for nourishing yin and is used in the deficiency syndrome of kidney and liver yin, which leads to a flare up of deficiency fire. The symptoms are tinnitus, night sweat, emission, hot flushes, dry mouth and throat. This syndrome is often seen in menopausal and post-menopausal women as well as diabetic patients.

It consists of three tonics and three purgatives. The three tonics are *shudihuang* (monarch), *shanzhuyu* (山茱萸) and *shanyao* (山药) (both are ministers). The three purgatives are *fuling, mudanpi* (牡丹皮) and *zexie* (泽泻). These three in combination play the adjuvant role of purging heat and removing dampness. There is no guiding herb.

Shudihuang nourishes kidney yin and essence, *shanzhuyu* enhances the action of nourishing kidney and liver yin, and *shanyao* strengthens spleen and reinforces the action of nourishing the kidney. The three purgative herbs reduce dampness, clear heat of yin deficiency, and enhance the transportation and transformation by the spleen. This is appropriate as the kidney is strongly dependent on the healthy functioning of the spleen to provide nutrients to the vital organs to sustain body activities.

Liuwei Dihuang Wan tonifies the kidney, liver and spleen as well as dissipates internal heat in a balanced and gentle manner. It is one of the most renowned and successful prescriptions in the history of Chinese medicine, used equally by physicians for treating illnesses, and by the common man as a dietary supplement to combat the weakening of the kidney functions that comes with stress and ageing.

Extensions: For strengthening kidney yang rather than yin, two warm herbs can be added to yield another classic formulation called the Pill for Nourishing Kidney Yang (*Shenqi Wan* 肾气丸). The added herbs *guizhi* (桂枝) and *fuzi* (附子) warm and invigorate the kidney. As the emphasis of the formulation has changed from nourishing yin to warming yang, the monarch herbs are the warm herbs *guizhi* and *fuzi*, and the *shudihuang* is the minister herb.

Another variation of this formulation known as *Jisheng Shenqi Wan* (济生肾气丸) is used in cases in which the deficiency of kidney yang has worsened and led to water retention. Diuretics such as *chuanniuxi* (川牛膝) and *cheqianzi* (车前子) are added to help excrete excess water from the body through urination. This prescription has been used by some physicians for treating urination difficulty due to benign prostate hyperplasia (enlargement).

The following are samples of formulations frequently used by physicians in clinical applications.

Erchen Tang (二陈汤)

This formulation is used for treating cough with wet phlegm due to the phlegm-dampness syndrome, with white sputum and thick white coating on the tongue. In this formulation, *banxia* (半夏) is the monarch herb and it targets the main syndrome by resolving phlegm and dampness. *Chenpi* (陈皮), the minister herb, enhances the action of *banxia* to remove phlegm and dampness. It also helps to regulate spleen qi since the presence of dampness and phlegm in the body tends to result in qi stagnation. *Fuling* is the adjuvant herb, strengthening the elimination of dampness through promoting urination, besides being also a mild spleen tonic. *Zhigancao*, the guiding herb, harmonizes the herbs in the formulation. The overall therapeutic actions are to resolve phlegm, eliminate dampness and promote qi flow.

Sini San (四逆散)

This formulation treats qi stagnation by regulating qi. Typical symptoms of qi stagnation are pain at the side of the rib cage, abdominal bloatedness (relieved after flatulence and burping), cold extremities and a taut pulse.

The four herbs in the formulation are *chaihu* (柴胡), the monarch, *baishao* (白芍) as minister, *zhishi* (枳实) as adjuvant, and *zhigancao* in the guiding role. *Chaihu* regulates liver qi to remove stagnation. *Baishao*, a blood tonic, nourishes blood in the liver to help it in qi regulation. *Zhishi* assists *chaihu* to enhance qi flow.

The spleen is often the first victim of qi stagnation, because of the over-restraint of the spleen by the liver, as the reader may recall in our discussions on *Wuxing* (the Five Element Model), which explains why *zhigancao*, a mild spleen tonic, is part of the formulation. *Extension*: Another variation of this formulation, used when qi stagnation worsens and affects blood flow, is *Chaihu Shugan San* (柴胡疏肝散) or "*Chaihu* Powder for Dredging the Liver". The symptoms presented can include depressive moods, chest tightness, severe abdominal distension and burping. Qi regulating herbs such as *xiangfu* (香附) and *chenpi* are used to further promote the qi flow of liver as well as the spleen. *Chenpi* also tonifies the spleen. Lastly, *chuanxiong* is added to promote qi and blood flow.

Xiaoyao San (逍遥散) or "Ease" Powder

The renowned Daoist philosopher *Zhuangzi* in his celebrated essay "Cruising at Ease" (*Xiaoyao You* 逍遥游) describes a mythical giant roc that flies at the speed of sound, cruising at ease without a care in the world, as implied by the title of the essay. The "ease" powder formulation borrows its name from *Zhuangzi's* allegory.

Xiaoyan San is prescribed for stagnation of liver qi and deficiency of blood and spleen arising from emotional stress affecting liver qi flow, which in turn suppresses the spleen function, causing digestive problems. The main symptom of this condition is moodiness, which explains the patient's need for "*xiaoyao*". It can be accompanied by headache, irregular menstruation, a taut pulse, and symptoms of weak spleen functions like poor appetite, lassitude and loose stools.

Xiaoyao San is in fact a variation of *Sini San*. *Danggui* and *baishao* are added as minister herbs to nourish liver blood and sustain the liver qi-dredging function. *Fuling* and *baizhu* are adjuvants fortifying the spleen against repression by the liver.

If the condition develops liver fire owing to prolonged stagnation of liver qi, heat-clearing herbs *mudanpi* (牡丹皮) and *zhizi* (栀子) are added to form *Danzhi Xiaoyaosan* (丹栀逍遥散) to help purge liver fire.

Decoctions for expelling blood stasis (*Zhuyu Tang* 逐瘀汤)

As the name suggests, this is a basic formulation for resolving blood stasis syndrome, characterized by stabbing pain and purplish/dark-coloured tongue. There are five different variations of the formulations, each targeting a different organ or location of blood stasis. The majority of these variations contain blood promoting and blood stasis resolving herbs such as *taoren, honghua* (usually as monarchs), *chuanxiong, chishao* (赤芍) (the ministers) and *danggui* (the adjuvant). The most commonly used *Zhuyu tang* is:

Decoction for Expelling Chest Blood Stasis (*Xuefu Zhuyu Tang* 血府逐瘀汤). Symptoms of chest blood stasis include localized chest stabbing pain, heart palpitation, insomnia, and dark-coloured lips with spots on the tongue. *Niuxi* (牛膝) (minister) is added to enhance the therapeutic effect of resolving blood stasis. *Shengdihuang* (生地黄), *zhiqiao* (枳壳) and *chaihu* (柴胡), as adjuvants, nourish liver yin and blood, and regulate the flow of liver qi. *Jiegeng* (桔梗) and *zhigancao* are the guiding herbs, with *jiegeng* directing the therapeutic effects to the chest and *zhigancao* harmonizing the actions of the herbs in the formulation.

Other formulations which follow similar principles of herbs combination are as follows. The name of the decoction indicates the part of the body that the decoction targets.

1) *Decoction for clearing orifices by improving blood flow (Tongqiao Huoxue Tang* 通窍活血汤)
2) *Decoction of expelling blood stasis below the diaphragm (Gexia Zhuyu Tang* 膈下逐瘀汤)
3) *Decoction of expelling blood stasis from the abdomen (Shaofu Zhuyu Tang* 少腹逐瘀汤)
4) *Decoction of expelling blood stasis from the body (Shengtong Zhuyu Tang* 身痛逐瘀汤)

Jade Screen Powder (*Yupingfeng San* 玉屏风散)

This formulation addresses deficiency in defensive qi characterized by profuse perspiration with aversion to wind, pale complexion and susceptibility to exogenous climatic pathogens especially wind. Its main therapeutic action is to replenish qi, especially defensive qi, and arrest perspiration. Individuals with this syndrome tend to have low *zhengqi* and catch colds or flu easily.

Huangqi (黄芪) is the monarch herb, replenishing qi and consolidating the outer layer of the body (superficies) against invasion of the exogenous pathogens. The minister herb *baizhu* tonifies qi by strengthening the spleen, which is the source of qi and blood production. *Fangfeng* (防风), the adjuvant herb, builds body resistance by expelling exogenous wind pathogens.

Pulse-activating Powder (*Shengmai Yin* 生脉饮)

Although this formulation arrests perspiration like Jade Screen Powder, it addresses a different form of perspiration, that of spontaneous sweating due to both qi and yin deficiency. Hence, it can be used in the treatment of chronic dry cough induced by qi and yin deficiency, with symptoms of breathlessness, fatigue, dryness in throat and profuse sweating day and night. Such conditions may be found in persons subjected to prolonged hot weather causing excessive perspiration, damaging the yin of the body and depleting its reserves of qi.

Ginseng, the monarch herb, addresses qi deficiency whereas the minister herb *maidong* (麦冬) nourishes yin to moisten the lung. *Wuweizi* (五味子), the adjuvant herb, encourages the production of fluids and arrests sweating to prevent excessive loss of body fluids.

Yinqiao San (银翘散)

This is a popular formulation for colds or flu induced by wind-heat pathogens, common in many tropical regions with a hot and humid climate. The invasion of the climatic wind-heat pathogens generally causes fever, chills, running nose, sore throat, headache, mild cough, and thirst. The patient has a red tongue and floating fast pulse.

The monarch herbs are the famous pair *yinhua* (银花) and *lianqiao* (连翘) for expelling wind-heat pathogens and clearing internal heat and toxins. There are two pairs of minister herbs. The first pair, peppermint leaves (薄荷) and *niubangzi* (牛蒡子), clear the head and soothe the throat; the second pair, *jingjie* (荆芥) and *dandouchi* (淡豆豉), enhance the effect of expelling the wind-heat pathogens. The adjuvants *lugen* (芦根) and *danzhuye* (淡竹叶) clear heat and promote production of fluids to quench thirst. *Jiegeng* is added to relieve cough. Raw *gancao* soothes the throat and also harmonizes the actions of all the herbs.

As this formulation is cool, it is not advisable for it to be taken long term as that could harm spleen and stomach qi.

Huoxiang Zhengqi San (藿香正气散)

This formulation is for stomach flu-like symptoms such as chills, fever, nausea, vomiting, diarrhoea, gastric and bloatedness with thick white fur on the tongue. It resolves syndromes arising from wind-cold pathogens and internal dampness that attack lung and spleen. Hence both diaphoretics with pungent-warm properties and herbs for resolving dampness are used in this warm-natured formulation.

The monarch herb *huoxiang* (藿香) uses strong pungent flavour to expel the wind-cold pathogens and resolves dampness from the spleen, hence alleviating nausea, vomiting, bloatedness and diarrhoea. The minister herbs include *banxia, chenpi, fuling* and *baizhu* resolve dampness and strengthen the spleen. The adjuvants *houpo* (厚朴) and *dafupi* (大腹皮) regulate qi flow in the spleen which stagnates because of dampness, thereby relieving abdomen bloatedness. Diaphoretics perillae leaf (紫苏叶) and *baizhi* (白芷) expel wind-cold pathogens, and *jiegeng* clears the lung. Ginger and red dates nourish the spleen. *Zhigancao* is the guiding herb. This formulation, which has a warm nature, is suitable for people whose tongues have thick white coating and experience diarrhoea and/or vomiting while overseas and encounter incompatibility of the local diet with their body constitutions. It is a useful medication to take with you when you travel.

How standard formulations are used in practice

In clinical practice, physicians would add or take off herbs from these formulations as adjustments to customize the prescription for the individual patient's condition.

For example, the standard formulation for treating flu due to external wind-heat syndrome is *Yinqiao San*. If the individual is also experiencing a bad sore throat and phlegmy cough in addition to the usual flu symptoms, an experienced TCM physician would consider adding herbs such as isatis root or *banlangeng* (板蓝根) and *zhebeimu* (浙贝母) into the formulation. Isatis root is a heat clearing herb that enhances the effect of soothing the throat and *zhebeimu* is stronger in resolving phlegm and relieving cough.

On the other hand, if the patient has a weak spleen and is suffering from flu of wind-heat syndrome, the physician would remove a few cooling herbs such as *lugen* and peppermint leaves and, at the same time, add some mild spleen qi tonics into the formulation. The purpose of making such adjustments is to protect the spleen whilst using the minimum number of heat clearing herbs in the original *Yinqiao San* formulation to expel external pathogens.

Chapter 8

Tonic Herbs and Recipes

TCM tonics are herbs for replenishing qi and blood, nourishing yin and yang, improving the functions of internal organs and body resistance to illness, and relieving various symptoms of weakness. Hence they are also known as restoratives (补虚药, 补益药). Tonics are mostly sweet in flavour and warm in nature, except for yin tonics which tend to be cool.

Chinese tonics are in a class of their own. There is probably no civilization that prizes tonics and makes use of them as much as the Chinese, who have a whole culture for using tonics to promote health, boost vitality and enhance longevity.

The judicious use of tonics needs good knowledge of the nature, properties and action of herbs. They cannot be indiscriminately used.

Guidelines on using tonics

1. Be clear about the deficiency syndrome for which tonics are being taken. Each category of tonic is used to address a different kind of deficiency syndrome. For example, *danggui* (当归) is usable for blood deficiency but not for yang deficiency. Ginseng can be used for either qi or yang deficiency syndrome, but not for yin deficiency.
2. Do not use tonics when you have an infection as that can aggravate the condition.
3. Tonics are more effective taken in small amounts over long periods of time. Excessive or wrong use of tonics can cause harm to the body.

4. Some tonics are difficult to digest, hence it is advisable to mix tonics with herbs such as Chinese yam (*shanyao* 山药) for strengthening the qi of the stomach and spleen and *chenpi* (陈皮) for improving the flow of qi.

8.1 Qi Tonics (补气药)

Most tonics are attributable to the spleen and lung meridians since the lung dominates qi and the spleen is the main source for qi production. It is used to treat qi deficiency syndrome manifested as fatigue, poor appetite, shortness of breath, weak pulse, and a pale tongue.

(i) Ginseng (*renshen* 人参)

Ginseng is the root of the *panax ginseng* plant and its use as a tonic goes back at least 4000 years. It is grown mainly in northeast of China. It is known as the "king of herbs" and "soil spirit" because of its legendary lifesaving effect. Nutrients in the soil are taken up by the ginseng plant, and after harvesting the soil can take up to 20 years to recover.

Therapeutic actions: Ginseng invigorates qi. Wild ginseng is reputed to have even stronger effect and is sometimes used in life-threatening situations when the patient is extremely weak from qi exhaustion.

Ginseng treats qi deficiency in the spleen, the heart and, in particular, the lung. It can improve coughs, shortness of breath and asthma due to lung qi deficiency. It is also an important herb for strengthening spleen qi, and can be used for treating fatigue, poor appetite and soft stools. It can also be used to calm the nerves for sounder sleep.

Ginseng also promotes production of fluids. It can be used to treat thirstiness due to loss of fluid during the recovery phase of febrile diseases or for diabetic patients who have qi deficiency and dryness.

Biomedical research suggests that ginseng can strengthen immunity, retard ageing, control blood glucose level, regulate the central nervous system and increase oxygen uptake in the heart.

Recipe: Ginseng wolfberry tea 人参枸杞茶

Ingredients: 3g sliced ginseng, 3g wolfberries
This tea is a tonic for health maintenance, especially for the elderly. Ginseng helps prevent premature deterioration of body functions while wolfberry tonifies the kidney to slow down ageing. Ginseng should not be taken with radish, which reduces its therapeutic effect.

Preparation method: Infuse in hot water and drink as a tea.

(ii) American ginseng (*xiyangshen* 西洋参)
This herb is native to North America but now widely cultivated in China. It is also known as *Huaqishen* (花旗参) and *Paoshen* (泡参).

Therapeutic actions: American ginseng is the only qi tonic that is cool in nature, hence it is suitable for people who lack qi and also have heat due to yin deficiency. This condition is common among people who burn the midnight oil and do not have enough rest, with symptoms of fatigue, spontaneous sweating, aversion to heat, thirst and scanty urine. American ginseng is good for clearing deficiency heat, but should not be used for excess heat with symptoms such has fever, red eyes, headache or giddiness.

Because the herb promotes production of fluid, it is used to treat patients who have exhausted qi and lost fluid often from a febrile condition that results in heavy sweating, diarrhoea or loss of blood.

Recipe: Noble Tea of Rejuvenation 君子复原茶

Ingredients: 3g American ginseng, 3g astragalus, 5g dendrobium, 3g wolfberries and 3 pieces red dates
Astragalus reinforces the qi tonifying effect of American ginseng, while dendrobium and wolfberry strengthen yin. Red date is a mild

qi tonic and gives a sweet taste to the tea. This tea is good for boosting energy and quenching thirst after a hot and tiring day.

Preparation method: Steep the ingredients in hot water for 10 minutes.

(iii) Codonopsis root (*dangshen* 党参)

This is a popular qi tonic with similar action as ginseng but weaker. It can be used as a substitute for ginseng when qi deficiency is mild. As it is more affordable, it has been called "the poor man's ginseng."

Therapeutic actions: Codonopsis root is used to treat spleen and lung qi deficiency with symptoms of body weakness, tiredness, poor appetite and soft stools. It can also tonify blood, hence it is suitable for qi and blood deficiency with symptoms like pale complexion, fatigue, light headedness, and heart palpitations. Codonopsis root also promotes fluid production, and is often used with yin tonics to treat qi and fluid lost due to heat.

Recipe: Pork liver porridge with codonopsis root and wolfberry 党参枸杞猪肝粥

Ingredients: 20g codonopsis root, 30g wolfberries, 50g pork liver (sliced into small pieces), 60g rice

This recipe is good for tonifying qi and blood. Pork liver replenishes blood. Wolfberry tonifies liver and kidney, which are organs that participate in the production and storage of blood. The liver opens into the eyes, hence this porridge is also good for nourishing the eyes.

Preparation method: Boil codonopsis root and wolfberry in a pot of water for 20 minutes, then use the pot of water to cook the rice. After the rice is almost cooked, put in the slices of pork liver.

(iv) Astragalus (*huangqi* 黄芪)

Astragalus or milkvetch, is known in Chinese as *huangqi* as well as *beiqi* (北芪). It is a very popular qi tonic and frequently used for cooking. The astragalus plant has long roots that can grow to 1.8m deep.

Therapeutic actions: Astraglaus strengthens defensive qi against external pathogens, whereas ginseng is stronger in tonifying the organs. It is the monarch herb in the prescription Jade screen powder (玉屏风散) which is useful for weak patients who are afraid of wind and sweat spontaneously.

Astragalus works well with diuretic herbs when treating water retention due to qi deficiency. It also helps in wound healing, and can be taken by patients after surgery.

When stir-baked with honey, astragalus becomes warmer in nature. This enhances its tonic effect for those with weak spleen qi characterized by poor appetite, fatigue and loose stools.

Recipe: Astragalus chicken soup 黄芪炖鸡汤

Ingredients: Half a chicken, 30g astragalus, 12 pieces red dates, 1.5 litres water

Chicken is a qi tonic food that synergizes well with astragalus. Red date has both qi and blood tonifying effects. Its sweetness helps make the soup delicious. As a light qi tonic soup, it is suitable for the whole family.

Preparation method: Put the herbs and chicken into a pot of 1.5 litres of water. Cook for 2 hours. Add salt for taste and serve warm.

(v) Chinese yam (*shanyao* 山药)

Chinese yam is the tuber of a species of flowering plant in the yam family. It is one of the four famous *Huai* herbs as it is cultivated largely in Henan province at an ancient location *Huai Qing Fu* (怀庆府). The Chinese yam that originates from there was also known as 怀山 or 淮山 (both pronounced as *huaishan*), or otherwise called *tiegun shanyao* (铁棍山药).

Chinese yam can be eaten raw and is used often as a tonic in medicated food as it is neutral (neither warm nor cool).

Therapeutic actions: Chinese yam is one of the top choices when treating gastrointestinal disorders. Although its spleen and stomach tonic effect may not be as strong as that of ginseng or codonopsis root, it is neutral and suitable for all ages as well as long term consumption.

Chinese yam also helps to tonify the lungs through the promotion effect of the five element principle, by which we tonify the lung through the spleen. It also helps with fluid production to nourish and moisturize the lung.

Chinese yam also tonifies the kidney and conserves essence and can be used to treat lower backache, frequent urination and urine incontinence. It is used to treat *xiaoke* (消渴), a condition similar to diabetes (see chapter 15).

Recipe: Chinese yam with strawberry sauce 草莓山药

Ingredients: 1 stick Chinese yam, strawberry, white vinegar, salt and sugar (amount based on personal taste)

This is a common appetizer in Chinese restaurants. The sweet and mildly sourish berries whets the appetite.

Preparation method: Cut the yam into short chunks. Dab yam chunks with vinegar to avoid oxidation then steam over medium to low heat for 20 minutes. Soak the strawberries in salted water for 10 minutes before removing the stalks and cutting them into small pieces. In a wok, add in 1 ladle of water and cut the strawberries. Stir and stew for about 15 minutes while adding some white sugar. After jam has thickened, take it out to cool. After the steamed yam has cooled, peel off the skin. Use a spoon to mash the yam. Mould the mashed yam into your desired serving shape, then pour the cooled strawberry jam over it.

(vi) Liquorice root (*gancao* 甘草)

Liquorice root is produced in Shanxi, Gansu and Xinjiang. It is often used as a harmonizer in herbal formulations.

Therapeutic actions: It is a mild and neutral qi tonic with mild pain relieving effect. It can help with abdominal cramps, heart palpitation and shortness of breath due to heart, spleen and stomach qi deficiency, and resolves phlegm from mild cough.

Liquorice as a qi tonic is used raw or honey-baked. Raw liquorice also clears heat and eliminates toxins and can be used for sore throat, boils, carbuncles and ulcers.

Liquorice should not be taken excessively or by itself for long periods of time as it contains glycyrrhizin which can cause side effects like high blood pressure, abnormal heart rhythm and water retention.

Recipe: Liquorice sour plum drink 甘草乌梅汤

Ingredients: 5g raw liquorice root, 15g smoked plums, rock sugar

During hot weather, qi is lost when there is excessive sweating. Liquorice strengthens qi and clears heat. With smoked plum, which promotes production of fluids, this makes a good drink to regain energy and quench thirst.

Preparation method: Add both herbs into a pot of water and boil for 5 minutes. After 5 minutes, remove the herbs. Add rock sugar to sweeten (optional).

(vii) Red date (*dazao* 大枣)

Chinese red date, known as jujube or jujuba, is the fruit of the plant *Ziziphus jujuba* harvested during autumn. As it ripens, it turns brown, but after sun-drying it wrinkles and turns dark purplish red.

Therapeutic actions: Red date warms and strengthens spleen qi, and is used for patients who are suffering from weakness, fatigue, loss of weight and loose stools. Because it tonifies blood and nourishes the heart to calm the mind, it can help with mild depression.

There are a few types of dates. While red dates are better with tonifying qi, candied red dates are good at strengthening spleen and stomach. Black dates (黑枣) and *nanzao* (南枣) are better at nourishing blood and tonifying liver and kidney.

Recipe: Chicken thigh red dates soup 鸡腿红枣汤

Ingredients: 2 chicken thighs, 12 red dates, 5 pieces dried mushrooms, 5g wolfberries, ginger and yellow wine, salt (to taste)

Chicken and mushrooms enhance the spleen qi strengthening effect of red dates. Wolfberry is a liver and kidney tonic and boosts the blood tonifying effect of the soup. Yellow wine helps to improve the flow of qi and blood.

Preparation method: Rinse and soak the mushrooms till they are soft. Put the chicken thighs, mushrooms, red dates and ginger into the pot. Pour in some yellow wine and water, then boil for about 45 minutes. Add salt to taste. Just before switching off the fire put in the wolfberries. Let the soup sit for 5 minutes before serving.

(viii) White hyacinth bean (*baibiandou* 白扁豆)

White hyacinth beans are the dried ripe seeds found in the thin pods of the *Dolicho lablab* L. plant. For medicinal purpose, they are dried in the sun and can be used either raw or after stir frying.

Therapeutic actions: White hyacinth bean tonifies the spleen and resolves dampness. Thus, it is used for digestive issues like poor appetite, nausea, vomiting, soft stools or diarrhoea, and excessive white discharge in women due to spleen qi deficiency. Raw white hyacinth beans are good for resolving dampness while the stir fried white hyacinth beans are better for tonifying the spleen.

Recipe: White hyacinth bean porridge 白扁豆粥

Ingredients: 15 to 50g white hyacinth bean, 3 to 10 pieces red dates, 50g rice

Porridges are easy to digest and have a mild qi tonifying effect which is enhanced with white hyacinth beans and red dates. As a mild qi tonic that is neutral in nature, this porridge is suitable for both children and the elderly with poor digestion.

Preparation method: Soak the white hyacinth bean for 2 hours. Cook the white hyacinth bean, rice and red dates in 3 bowls of water. After it boils, continue cooking for 30 to 45 minutes until the porridge is soft.

(ix) Rhodiola rosea (*hongjingtian* 红景天)

Rhodiola rosea is a perennial plant that grows at high altitudes and harsh environments; it is also used as medicine for coping with high altitude stress and sickness.

Therapuetic actions: Tonifies qi and clears the lungs; useful for weak spleen qi symptoms like fatigue, lethargy and lung yin deficiency cough with sticky phlegm. As this herb improves blood circulation and reduces blood stasis, it can be combined with other blood promoting herbs to treat bruises resulting from trauma and injury.

Recipe: Rhodiola rosea black chicken soup 红景天乌鸡汤

Ingredients: 10 to 20g rhodiola rosea, one black chicken, 2 pieces red dates , salt, white pepper, ginger, spring onion (to taste)

This soup is good for people who tire easily. Cooked with black chicken, it has qi and blood tonifying effect. The addition of red dates enhances the qi tonifying effect and gives the soup a sweet taste.

Preparation method: Soak the rhodiola rosea for 20 minutes in a cooking pot before adding black chicken, red dates, ginger and spring onions. Add enough water to cover all ingredients. Bring to a boil, after which reduce fire and continue to boil for another 2 hours.

8.2 Yang Tonics (补阳药)

These are mainly attributed to the kidney meridian, the kidney being the main source of body yang. Yang tonics are used to treat kidney yang deficiency manifested in cold limbs, backaches, and male sexual dysfunction. They are mostly sweet, pungent and salty in flavour and warm in nature.

(i) Eucommia bark (*duzhong* 杜仲)

Widely cultivated and highly valued in China because of the medicinal use of its bark, the eucommia tree must be at least 10 years old for its bark to be harvested.

Therapeutic actions: Eucommia bark is used for liver and kidney deficiency manifested in bone and tendon symptoms like lower backache and knee weakness. Kidney deficiency may also cause premature ageing, tinnitus, hearing loss, and frequent urination as well as erectile dysfunction in men and menstrual or miscarriage issues in women.

Recipe: Eucommia bark chicken feet soup 杜仲鸡脚汤

Ingredients: 8 pieces chicken feet, 250g chestnut, 20g eucommia bark, 3g dried tangerine peel

This soup is good for people with lower back ache due to kidney deficiency. Chicken feet nourish tendons and bones, chestnuts tonify the kidney, and tangerine peels give the soup a pleasant aroma besides helping with the flow of spleen qi for digestion.

Preparation method: Put the ingredients in a pot and add water, bring to boil, then turn to medium heat and continue boiling for 2 hours.

(ii) Himalayan Teasel Root (*xuduan* 续断)

The Himalayan teasel root, well known for healing fractures, is called *xuduan* (续断) in Chinese, which means connect the broken. It is also called *chuanduan* (川断) as it is mainly grown in Sichuan. The root has very similar therapeutic value to eucommia bark and the two herbs are often used as a pair (药对).

Therapeutic actions: Tonifying kidney and liver, strengthening and repairing bones and tendons, and preventing miscarriages and heavy menstrual bleeding.

Recipe: Pig's tail soup 猪尾汤

Ingredients: 400g pig's tail , 25g himalayan teasel root, 30g eucommia bark, salt (to taste)

Pig's tail is rich in collagen and tonifies the kidney, strengthens the lower back and nourishes bone marrow. Cooked together with the two herbs, the soup strengthens the kidney and lower back, and is good for pregnant women by preventing miscarriages.

Preparation method: Remove hair from the pig's tail, cut it into chunks and blanch in hot water. Put the rinsed herbs in a filter bag, add to the rest of the ingredients and water in a pot. Bring to boil before lowering the fire to simmer for about 40 minutes, or cook until the pig's tail meat is soft. Add salt to flavour.

(iii) Cordyceps (*dongchong xiacao* 冬虫夏草)

Cordyceps, also known as caterpillar fungus, grow from fungus that lives in the larvae of ghost moths. As the fungus germinates in the living larvae, it eventually kills and mummifies it. A dark brown stalk-like body emerges and stands upright. Cordyceps are mainly found in meadows above 4000 meters in the Himalayan regions of Nepal, Bhutan, India and Tibet. Good quality cordyceps are those with big full worm body and short fungi stalk. They can be very expensive as they are getting rarer with strong demand from East Asian consumers.

Therapeutic actions: Cordyceps enjoy a good reputation in Chinese households as a tonic for treating asthma, chronic coughs and slow recovery during convalescence. The lung governs respiratory qi and kidney original qi. As it can tonify both lung and kidney, resolve phlegm and stop bleeding, cordycep is used to treat asthma and chronic coughs with phlegm or blood. As a kidney yang tonic it can also be used to treat erectile dysfunction and night emission due to kidney deficiency.

Recipe: Cordyceps and black bean soup 虫草黑豆汤

Ingredients: 2 to 3 pieces cordyceps, 150g lean meat, 50g black beans, 3 pieces red dates, 5 pieces dried longan

Black beans are nutritious kidney tonic foods that promote blood circulation and diuresis. They also expel wind and eliminate toxins. Black beans and cordyceps tonify the kidney, while red dates and longan tonify qi and blood. This soup is good for chronic respiratory illnesses and slow convalescence.

Preparation method: Rinse the black beans and soak for 2 hours. Brush away the soil and wash the cordyceps, and rinse the red dates and dried longan. Cut the meat into cubes and blanch in hot water. Put the black beans, dried longan and meat into a clay pot. Boil for 2 hours. Add cordyceps and boil for another 30 minutes, followed by red dates for another 15 minutes. Add salt to taste.

8.3 Blood Tonics (补血药)

Blood tonics are used to treat blood deficiency with symptoms such as pale lips, complexion, and nails, dizziness, palpitations, delayed menstruation, and insomnia. These are mainly attributed to the heart and liver meridians, which is consistent with the heart governing blood and the liver storing blood.

(i) Chinese angelica root (*danggui* 当归)

Chinese angelica root tonifies and regulates the flow of blood to ensure that blood is well distributed to the different parts of the body. Hence, in Chinese it is also known as *danggui* (当归) which means to return blood to its rightful place. The head and the body of the root have stronger effect in nourishing blood whereas the tail is better for promoting blood flow.

Therapeutic actions: The Chinese angelica root tonifies blood. As it also regulates menstruation, it is often used to treat women's health issues, hence it has been called the "female ginseng", although men with blood deficiency can equally use it. Its action of promoting blood flow and relieving pain due to poor blood flow makes it useful for the treatment of abdominal pain, trauma and injuries. The

Chinese angelica root has oil constituents to help nourish the large intestine to relieve constipation due to dry stools.

Recipe: Danggui egg 当归鸡蛋

Ingredients: An egg, 10g Chinese angelica root, 5 pieces red dates, 3 pieces dried longan, brown sugar

Red dates and longan enhance the blood tonifying effect of the Chinese angelica root. The addition of the brown sugar, which also tonifies and promotes the flow of blood, gives the soup a slight sweetness. For women, this dish can be taken for better complexion and also after menstruation to replenish blood.

Preparation method: Boil the eggs till they are cooked and deshell. Put the eggs together with *danggui*, red dates and longan in a pot of water. Bring to boil, then reduce to small fire and continue to cook for another 30 minutes. 5 minutes before turning off the fire, add brown sugar.

(ii) Processed Rehmannia Root (*shudihuang* 熟地黄)

Rehmannia root, known as the "Chinese foxglove", is also one of the famous four *Huai* herbs. Depending on how it is being processed, the therapeutic actions of the rehmannia roots differ. The fresh rehmannia root mainly clears heat and cools the blood while the dried rehmannia root cools the blood and also nourishes yin. Processed rehmannia root is slightly warm and has the blood tonifying effect. Processing consists of nine cycles of steaming and sun drying.

Therapeutic actions: Processed rehmannia root tonifies blood and nourishes yin, which is essential for the production of blood. It also supplements kidney essence and marrow and is a component of formulations for treating delayed growth in children, reproduction issues (low sex drive and infertility) and premature ageing. Processed rehmannia root and Chinese angelica root are a good pair for mutual reinforcement as blood tonics.

Recipe: Rehmannia root and black chicken soup 熟地黑鸡汤

Ingredients: Black chicken (cut into small pieces), 9g processed rehmannia root, 9g dried rehmannia root, 4g *chuanxiong*, 12g astragalus, 12g red dates, 6g wolfberry, salt (to taste)

Black chicken is a usual choice of meat for medicated blood tonic food. Dried rehmannia root mitigates the warm nature of the soup while processed rehmannia is the main herb to tonify blood. *Chuanxiong* and astragalus are added to promote blood flow and supplement qi to help with the production of blood. Red dates and wolfberry are added for taste, but also play roles in tonifying qi and kidney respectively. As this soup tonifies both blood and kidney, it is suitable for people with reproduction issues and premature ageing.

Preparation method: Rinse all the herbs (except wolfberry) and put them in a filter bag. Next, soak the bag of herbs in a pot of 1.5 litre of water for 20 minutes before cooking. Cook the herbs for 30 minutes before putting in the black chicken and cook for another 1.5 to 2 hours. Add wolfberry and salt before turning off the fire. Stir well and serve.

(iii) *Ejiao* (阿胶)
Ejiao in processed form looks like translucent brownish tiles. It is in fact hardened gelatin extracted from the skin of donkeys by a process of soaking and stewing. Because of its high nutritional value, it was used as tribute to the imperial family in China for health and beauty enhancement.

Therapeutic actions: *Ejiao* tonifies blood and nourishes yin. It is especially good for blood deficiency syndrome due to blood loss, and is also used to stop bleeding. It can be ground into powder, and taken when there is abnormal uterine bleeding, blood in urine during pregnancy, or nose bleeds. As it nourishes yin and moistens the lung, it sometimes can be used to treat dry coughs with scanty or blood-streaked phlegm. As a tonic, *ejiao* is used in beauty enhancement and strengthening muscles and tendons, and generally improving health.

Recipe: Ejiao paste 阿胶膏

Ingredients: 125g *ejiao*, 240ml yellow wine, 60g rock sugar (to taste)
Yellow wine is used to dissolve the gelatin. It also improves blood circulation, thus enabling *ejiao* to tonify blood without introducing stasis.

Preparation method: Crush the gelatine into smaller pieces then soak it in yellow wine for 1 to 3 days in a clay pot. After the *ejiao* has dissolved, add icing sugar. Steam the pot for 1 hour, stirring the pot every 20 minutes. After it cools down, store in a refrigerator and mix with milk or water.

(iv) Root of tuber fleeceflower (*heshouwu* 何首乌)
The root of tuber fleeceflower is a revitalising herb used as a tonic to slow down ageing and promote hair growth. Legend has it that a man with the surname of '*He*' (何) had a dream about this root, and later actually found it. After ingesting the herb, his grey hair turned black and he lived to the age 160. This root has mild toxicity, hence it is advisable not to take a high dosage and for a prolonged period.

Therapeutic actions: The unprocessed root eliminates toxin of carbuncles and boils, treats malaria and promotes bowel movement. After processing by steaming with black beans juice and wine, it tonifies essence and blood. TCM believes that lustrous hair indicates abundant blood supply (发为血之余). Hence, processed *heshouwu* helps hair growth and prevents premature greying through tonifying blood. As it is also a kidney and liver tonic, it helps to strengthen muscle and tendon, slows down ageing and is helpful for treating infertility.

Recipe: Root of tube fleeceflower tea 首乌茶

Ingredients: 10g processed root of tuber fleeceflower, 10g processed rehmannia root, 5g honey-baked liquorice

Both herbs tonify blood and kidney essence and make a good pair for promoting hair growth. Liquorice tonifies qi and gives a sweet taste to the tea.

Preparation method: Rinse the herbs then infuse them in hot water for 15 minutes.

8.4 Yin Tonics (补阴药)

Yin tonics are mainly attributed to the kidney, liver, lung and stomach meridians. Most are slightly cool in nature, which suit yin deficiency heat symptoms. Typical yin deficiency symptoms are dryness in the mouth, throat and skin, hot flashes, tinnitus, and lower back soreness. Yin deficiency people easily get hungry but eat with no weight gain, and have a red tongue with thin fur.

(i) Root of coastal glehnia (*beishashen* 北沙参)
Beishashen is from the root of the plant *Glehnia littoralis* from the carrot family, named coastal glehnia as it grows along the coast. The leaves look like corals and are eaten as vegetables by the Chinese and Koreans. The roots are used as a yin tonic. Closely related is the fourleaf ladybell root (*nanshashen* 南沙参), found mostly in southern China, hence "*nan*" to indicate its southern origin.

Therapeutic actions: *Beishashen* nourishes lung yin and clears lung heat. It is used to treat dry coughs during autumn and those who spend a lot of time in dry air-conditioned rooms. It also nourishes stomach yin and promotes production of fluid, making it suitable for stomach yin deficiency with symptoms of thirstiness, hunger with poor appetite, abdominal pain and dry stools.

Nanshashen has the same therapeutic value as *beishashen* but is less potent, hence the latter is used more widely as medicine. *Nanshashen* also tonifies qi and resolves phlegm.

Recipe: Shashen white fungus drink 银耳沙参饮

Ingredients: 30g white fungus, 20g *beishashen*, 10g wolfberries, 50g rock sugar (to taste), 1 litre water

White fungus, used as a vegetable or in desserts, is neutral and nourishes yin. Combined with *beishashen* and wolfberry, this drink works well to nourish lung yin and relieve dry cough.

Preparation method: Soak the white fungus for 1 hour, during which change the water at least twice. Next, remove the yellowish hard base. Meanwhile, rinse the *beishashen* and soak it for 20 minutes. Put the white fungus, *beishashen* and water into a pot and bring to boil. Reduce heat and continue to boil for another 1 hour. 5 minutes before turning off the fire, add wolfberry and rock sugar.

(ii) Dwarf lilyturf tuber (*maidong* 麦冬)

Dwarf lilyturf is an evergreen perennial plant that bears a distinctive blue berry fruit. It is a hardy plant and can survive temperatures of −20°C, and grows well under sun or partial shade. *Maidong*, tuberous root of this plant, is used as a yin tonic. Some varieties of *maidong* have cores and others do not. It is believed that those with cores are better as they not only nourish yin but also clear heart fire.

Therapeutic actions: *Maidong* is used to treat yin deficiency with heat in the lung and stomach with symptoms like dry cough with little phlegm, dry throat, thirst, abdominal pain, hunger, dry stools and constipation. In addition, it clears deficiency heat in the heart, and may help insomnia with vivid dreams, irritable moods and heart palpitations.

Recipe: Nourishing yin duck soup 养阴鸭汤

Ingredients: 30g *beishashen*, 30g *nanshashen*, 30g *maidong*, 30g solomonseal rhizome (玉竹), half a duck, spring onion, ginger, yellow wine, salt

The four herbs used in this soup tonify yin and promote fluid production. Duck meat is also a yin tonic and is the common meat of choice for medicated yin tonic food. Spring onion, ginger and yellow wine reduce duck meat odour.

Preparation method: Wash the duck and remove the excess fat. Rinse the herbs and soak them in water for about 20 minutes then put them and the duck in a pot of water. Bring it to boil and continue to cook at high heat for about 10 minutes. Remove the layer of fat on the surface of the water and add yellow wine, spring onion and ginger. Reduce fire and boil till the duck is cooked. Add salt to taste.

(iii) Dendrobium (*shihu* 石斛)

Dendrobium belongs to the orchid family and bears beautiful flowers of ornamental value. "*Shi*" means rock, and dendobrium is named *shihu* as the wild dendrobium "lives on the rocks." There are more than a thousand species of dendrobium but only a few are used in Chinese medicine. The part of the plant that is used as a herb is the matured stem of the plant, which is dried and usually curled up into small compact balls for storage.

Therapeutic actions: Dendrobium tonifies stomach yin and promotes the production of fluid. It is used in the treatment of febrile disease and diabetes when the patient demonstrates excessive thirst. It also clears deficiency heat to alleviate dry cough, night sweats and low-grade fever. Dendobrium is known to improve vision, partly because it moisturises dry eyes, but also because it tonifies the kidney, which strengthens the liver through the five-element principle. (The eyes are "the opening orifices of the liver.")

Recipe: Dendrobium chrysanthemum tea 石斛菊花茶

Ingredients: 10g dendrobium, 3g wolfberry, 5g chrysanthemum, 1 piece candied red date, 800ml water

This drink is good for dry eyes symptom. Dendrobium and wolfberry are often used as a pair to tonify liver and kidney so as to improve vision. Chrysanthemum clears liver heat to clear the eyes. Candied red date is added to strengthen the spleen and stomach, as well as to give the drink a light sweet taste.

Preparation method: Rinse the dendrobium, wolfberry and chrysanthemum. Soak them in 800 ml of water for 20 minutes. Add the candied red date and boil for about 15 minutes.

(iv) Lily Bulb (*baihe* 百合)

The lily bulb is a vegetable that looks similar to garlic. When used fresh, it has a crunchy texture and sweet taste. However, for medical use, the lily bulb is usually prepared and dried for storage.

Therapeutic actions: The lily bulb nourishes and moistens the lungs to help with dry cough. It can also clear heat in the heart and calm the mind, hence improves sleep.

Recipe: Steamed lily bulb 蒸百合

Ingredients: 200g fresh lily bulb , 20g honey or brown sugar
This is a simple recipe which can be served as a dessert in the evening, and calms the mind for better sleep.

Preparation method: Coat the lily bulb pieces with honey or sugar then steam.

(v) Solomonseal rhizome (*yuzhu* 玉竹)

The Solomonseal rhizome is a common herbal ingredient for home-cooked herbal soup. It gives the soup a pleasant sweet taste. It is slightly cold in nature and thus suitable for warm climates like that of Singapore.

Therapeutic actions: It nourishes yin and moistens dryness, and is used for lung yin deficiency with symptoms like dry cough, hoarse voice, dry throat and blood-streaked phlegm. *Yuzhu* also improves poor appetite due to stomach yin deficiency. Used with *maidong*, it can nourish heart yin and clear heat to relieve irritability, anxiety, and excess perspiration.

Recipe: Yuzhu sea coconut soup 玉竹海底椰汤

Ingredients: 20g *yuzhu*, 20g *beishashen*, 3 pieces dried fig, 5 pieces sea coconut, 200g pork shank, 1.5 litres water, salt

This soup is suitable for people with dry cough and little phlegm. Sea coconut and figs nourish the lungs to relieve cough. With the addition of two herbs, the lungs are further nourished and moistened, and fluid production improved to relieve thirst and dryness. This soup may not be suitable for people with chesty coughs and yellow phlegm.

Preparation method: Blanch the pork shank in boiling water for 5 minutes. Put the herbs, blanched pork, dried figs and sea coconut in a pot of 1.5 litres of water. Bring to boil over medium high heat. After that, cook over low heat for 1 hour. Add salt to taste.

(vi) Wolfberry (*gouqizi* 枸杞子)

Wolfberry, also known as goji berry, originates from Ningxia, China. It is the beautiful red fruit of the *Lycium barbarum* plant. In recent years, wolfberry and its derived products have gained popularity as health foods. Biomedical research suggests that the wolfberry also has functions like anti-ageing, lowering blood glucose and improving immunity.[12]

Therapeutic actions: Wolfberry is one of the few yin tonics that is neutral in nature. It tonifies kidney and liver yin and treats premature ageing conditions like hearing and hair loss, premature greying, loose teeth, insomnia and infertility. Wolfberry is also known to improve vision as it tonifies kidney essence.

Recipe: Dendrobium chrysanthemum tea 石斛菊花茶
　　See earlier entry on dendrobrium.

　　Wolfberry is believed to be best eaten raw, as steeping or boiling of wolfberry may not allow its effective compounds to be fully released into the water. However, the Chinese are very used to having some of it in their soups for tonifying as well as visual presentation of the dish. It is advised to add in the wolfberries 15 minutes before the soups are served so as to retain most of its useful ingredients.

---

[12] Sun *et al* (2021)

(vii) Mulberry fruit (*sangshen* 桑椹)

The fruit of the mulberry tree can be eaten fresh or dried. It can be made into wine, fruit juice, or a jam, and even a snack. It is very nutritious, high in vitamin C, iron, and anthocyanins.[13] It is also rich in dietary fibre and thus improves digestion.

Therapeutic actions: The mulberry fruit nourishes yin and also tonifies blood. It is used to treat giddiness, tinnitus, poor vision, joint stiffness, insomnia and premature greying of hair due to liver and kidney yin deficiency. It promotes production of fluid, hence helps with dryness syndrome with symptoms like thirst, constipation and dry stools.

Recipe: Mulberry longan red dates paste 桑椹桂圆红枣膏

Ingredients: 1.2kg fresh mulberries , 20g longan meat, 10g red dates, honey (optional)

This paste can be eaten as a spread on bread, or mixed with water as a health drink to tonify the kidney. Longan meat and red dates enhance the blood tonifying function of the mulberry and also neutralise the cold nature of the mulberry fruit, thus making the paste suitable even for people with weak stomachs.

Preparation method: Blend the mulberries, filter out the fruit pulps from the juice and keep them aside. Put the mulberry juice, longan meat and red dates into a pot. Cook the juice until one third of the juice is left. Put the mulberry fruit pulp back into the juice. Add honey to thicken the mixture.

(viii) Black sesame seed (*heizhima* 黑芝麻)

Black sesame seeds are small, flat, oily seeds that grow in the fruit pods of the *Sesamum indicum* plant. They are highly valued for anti-ageing and promoting longevity. The *Compendium of Materia Medica* (*Bencao Gangmu* 本草纲目) documents: "Consuming black

---

[13] Anthocyanins are colored water-soluble pigments belonging to the phenolic group. They contain antioxidants.

sesame for a hundred days can cure all chronic ailments. After a year facial complexion will be glowing; in the second year grey hairs return to black; in the third, teeth will become stronger."

Black sesame seed is also a good source of protein and minerals such as iron, zinc, copper and magnesium. However, because it is high in fibre and rich in oils, it has a mild laxative effect and is not recommended for people with chronic diarrhoea.

Therapeutic actions: Neutral in nature, it tonifies kidney essence and nourishes liver blood and is often used with other kidney tonics to treat ageing-related problems like giddiness, poor vision, premature greying of hair and limb weakness. As it is rich in oil, it can lubricate the intestines and treat constipation due to blood deficiency.

The white (hulled) sesame seeds have similar medical benefits as the black seeds, but the former is better for moistening the large intestine and skin, while the latter is better for tonifying kidney and liver.

Recipe: Black sesame paste 芝麻糊

Ingredients: 250g black sesame seeds , 50g glutinous rice, 2 teaspoons granulated sugar or rock sugar, 1 teaspoon salt, 400ml water

This is a popular and famous Chinese dessert. It is tasty and nutritious and may be taken regularly.

Preparation method: Soak glutinous rice for at least 5 hours. Fry the black sesame seeds in a pan over low heat till there is sizzling sound, tossing and stirring to prevent burning. Leave aside to cool. Add the sesame seeds, glutinous rice and 200ml of water into a blender. Blend till it is smooth. Filter the blend and remove the fibres. Boil 200ml of hot water in a pot and add the sesame mix to the hot water. Add sugar and salt, and continue to let it simmer until it is thickened.

8.5 General Tonics

Ganoderma lucidum (lingzhi 灵芝*)*

Ganoderma lucidum is an oriental fungus with legendary power for promoting health and longevity, and is popular in China, Japan, and other Asian countries. It is a large, dark mushroom with a glossy exterior and a woody texture. In Chinese, the name *lingzhi* represents spiritual power and essence of immortality, and is regarded as the "herb of spiritual potency."[14]

Lingzhi has become a prized health supplement because of its claimed medical benefits. It has also been exotically described as a tonic for the three treasures of qi, essence (*jing*) and spirit (*shen*). *Lingzhi* and its cousin *yunzhi* (云芝) are used for complementary treatment of cancer patients. Limited scale biomedical research suggests that it strengthens the immune system and may have anti-cancer effects. In Chinese folklore, *lingzhi* is a herb that can be taken long term to slow ageing and enhance longevity.

Therapeutic actions: Lingzhi is attributable to the heart, kidney, liver and lung meridians. In mainstream TCM, *lingzhi* is regarded primarily as a calmative and a qi tonic. It is useful for heart qi deficiency with symptoms like heart palpitation, forgetfulness and body weaknesses. As a calmative, it aids sleep but also sharpens mind focus when awake. It helps to warm the lungs to resolve wet phlegm and relieve cough or asthma and may be suitable for people with chronic fatigue.

Recipe: Pork rib soup with Chinese yam and lingzhi (淮山灵芝排骨汤)

Ingredients: Pork ribs (blanched with hot water), 3 to 4 pieces *lingzhi*, 20 to 30 pieces red dates (seeds removed), fresh Chinese yam

---

[14] Wachtel-Galor, S *et al* (2011)

(skinned, cut into small pieces), 4 to 5 pieces dendrobium, salt to taste

With pork, *lingzhi*, red dates and Chinese yam, the soup is a mild qi and blood tonic. With the addition of dendrobium, it tonifies the kidney and strengthens the various functions of the kidney.

Preparation method: Add pork ribs, *lingzhi*, red dates and dendrobium into a pot of water. Cook for 30 minutes to soften the pork ribs. Add Chinese yam and continue to cook for 20 to 25 minutes. Add salt to taste.

Chapter 9

Herbs and Recipes for Clearing External Pathogens

Diaphoretics are a group of herbs that clear external pathogens from the body through perspiration. External pathogens, also known as climatic pathogens, invade the body through the skin, inducing "external" syndromes, manifested in flu-like symptoms such as chills, body aches, running nose, cough and a floating pulse.

You may be pleased to know that most of the diaphoretics are everyday ingredients in your kitchen such as ginger, spring onion and coriander. They can commonly be identified by their strong pungent smell. Generally, diaphoretics should only be cooked for 5 to 10 minutes as the active components are volatile and the high heat can reduce their strong pungent flavour.

Diaphoretics are divided into two categories, namely the pungent warm and pungent cool herbs.

9.1 Diaphoretics with Pungent Warm Properties (辛温解表药)

This group of diaphoretics is warm in nature hence is used to treat external wind cold syndrome with symptoms such as sneezing, aversion to cold and wind, runny and clear mucus, slight cough, fever, and light red tongue with thin white fur.

(i) Perillae leaf (*zisu* 紫苏)
The next time when you dine in at a Japanese restaurant, take a closer look at the green purplish leaves that your sashimi sits on. These leaves are not there for decorative purposes but to be eaten

with the sashimi to remove toxins and mitigate the cold nature of raw fish. The greenish purple herb is perillae leaf, which is also known as the shiso leaf in Japan or Chinese basil because of its strong fragrance. These leaves either come in full green colour or one side green and the underside purple. Both the fresh and dried forms can be used for cooking although the dried ones are often used in medical formulations.

Therapeutic actions: The perillae leaf can expel wind cold pathogens and also regulate abdominal qi which tends to stagnate because of cold pathogens. In addition, perillae leaf helps to detoxify seafoods.

If one experiences nausea, vomiting and bloated stomach after eating foods or drinks that are cold in nature such as sashimi and seafoods, perillae leaf can be used to alleviate these symptoms. The herb is safe to use in pregnant women, especially for those who are in the first trimester experiencing nausea, vomiting and bloating as it regulates spleen qi without destabilizing pregnancy.

Recipe: Tomatoes soaked with perilla leaves 紫苏浸番茄

Ingredients: 5 pieces of fresh perilla leaves (preferably those that are purple in colour), 10 cherry tomatoes (preferably those on the vine), 100g honey, 2 teaspoon sugar, 3 to 4 pieces of smoked plums (*wumei* 乌梅). 1 small bowl of white wine is optional

Tomatoes nourish the stomach to improve appetite and promote the production of fluids to quench thirst. Perillae leaf is added not only to regulate the spleen qi but also to mitigate the cool nature of the tomatoes so that this dish is not too cooling for the spleen. Smoked plums are added to enhance the action of promoting the production of fluids. Together with the sweet tangy sauce, this dish is a good appetizer and suitable for individuals suffering from a bloated stomach.

Preparation method: Boil the smoked plums in water for around 20 to 30 minutes. Set aside the water. Wash the cherry tomatoes and peel off the skin (Soak the tomatoes in warm water to facilitate easy removal of skin). After removing the skin, put the cherry tomatoes in ice water to make the tomatoes firmer. Sauce: mix the honey, sugar, white wine (optional), plum water and perilla leaves together. Soak the tomatoes in the sauce for 2 hours.

(ii) Fresh ginger (*shengjiang* 生姜)

Ginger is very commonly used in cooking and most people know about its effect of expelling wind, especially from the abdomen. Ancients have used it and is believed that Confucius ate it every day and lived to a ripe old age. Ginger is also used in many Chinese medical formulations.

Therapeutic actions: When we are exposed to cold or rain, a warm cup of ginger drink can make us feel better. The warmth and pungent flavour of the ginger drink not only helps to expel the wind cold pathogens from the lung but also from the spleen and stomach. Therefore, it can be used to treat cough, running nose and watery clear phlegm resulting from external wind cold syndrome.

Ginger is also known as the panacea for vomiting (呕家之圣药) because of its effectiveness in alleviating nausea due to cold pathogens in the spleen and stomach by causing stomach qi to descend. Like the perillae leaf, it can also be used in pregnant women for morning sickness without endangering pregnancy.

A favourite ingredient for cooking fish, ginger is well known for its ability to reduce unpleasant "fishy" odours. This is attributed to its pungent flavour and anti-bacterial properties which enable it to mildly detoxify foods.

Recipe: Ginger tea with perillae leaves 生姜紫苏饮

Ingredients: 3g of ginger, 15g of red sugar, 3g of perillae leaves

The combination of ginger and perilla leaves make this a perfect tea for relieving nausea and bloated stomach and preventing of colds after exposure to cold and rainy weather. Red sugar has a warm nature and assists the ginger and perillae leaves to expel the wind cold pathogens. The sweetness of red sugar also helps to soften the pungent taste of ginger and perillae leaves to make the tea more palatable. Individuals with a heaty body constitution should avoid drinking this tea.

Preparation method: Chop the ginger into thin slices and break the perillae leaves into small pieces. Add red sugar and hot water. Cover and simmer for 10 minutes. Serve warm.

(iii) Chinese green onion (*congbai* 葱白)

This long leafy vegetable with a short white bulb at the bottom is used as garnish in cooking. It is also known as spring onion or scallion. The green portion of the green onion is used in cooking. However, the white bulb has the most medicinal value, even though it is usually discarded. This part has a stronger pungent flavour. A good quality green onion is characterised by greener leaves and longer white bulb.

Therapeutic actions: In Chinese medicine, the bulb of the green onion is used in prescriptions. Compared to the other diaphoretics, it is weaker in expelling wind cold pathogens, hence its use in milder conditions of colds and flu.

The warm nature of the Chinese green onion improves the flow of yang qi in the body by dispelling cold pathogens that can cause abdominal pain and difficulty in urination. This is usually done by pounding the green onion and applying it warm on the navel. When the pounded green onion is applied externally on breasts, it can help to relieve engorgement by unblocking the milk ducts and promoting lactation. In addition, green onion can be used to kill parasites and remove toxins, which explains its application for swollen carbuncles and ulcers.

Recipe: Green onion chicken soup 葱白鸡汤

Ingredients: 3 bunches of green onions (chopped), 1 chicken thigh (deboned). Salt and white pepper are optional.

This is a soul-warming soup for those with a cold or mild flu with weak appetite resulting from wind cold pathogens (for example, through being caught in the rain). It should be consumed hot to induce sweating.

Preparation method: Boil 1 bowl of water. Without using oil, pan fry the chicken thigh using the fats from the skin over low heat until the skin is golden brown. Cut the chicken thigh into strips. Pour out the chicken oil from the pan and stir fry the chicken until it is cooked. Pour boiled water into the pan. Season it with salt and white pepper to taste. Cook the chicken soup until it is boiling. Pour into a bowl of chopped spring onions. Serve warm.

(iv) Coriander leaves (*husui* 胡荽)

Coriander leaves, also known as cilantro and Chinese parsley, are used as a garnish in Asian cooking. They have a peculiar taste and smell that some people do not like. However, it is these strong diaphoretic properties that make them valuable as medicine.

Therapeutic actions: Like Chinese green onion, coriander leaves have a weaker action in expelling wind cold pathogens, hence they are usually used with other diaphoretics.

Before the 21st century when measles and chicken pox were prevalent in many countries, coriander leaves were used to provide relief from these infectious diseases by releasing toxins from the body. This can be done by steaming and washing the body with boiled coriander leaves water.

Although some people are put off by the smell of coriander leaves, there are people whose appetites improve with them, especially those who have bloated stomachs from foods that are cold in nature. The strong fragrance of the coriander leaves "awakens" the spleen and stomach and promotes its qi flow.

The fragrance of the coriander leaves needs to be retained in order for its therapeutic actions to be effective, which explains why we tend to eat them raw or cook them for a short period of time.

Recipe: Coriander leaf omelette 胡荽煎蛋

Ingredients: 3 stalks of fresh coriander, 4 thin slices of ginger with skin removed, 3 eggs, 1 teaspoon sesame oil, ¼ teaspoon white pepper powder, a pinch of salt (optional)

This simple and tasty recipe improves digestion and relieves a bloated stomach. Eggs nourish the stomach and spleen, and ginger is added to enhance the effect of regulating the spleen qi. With this combination of ingredients, this dish may even win over the tastebuds of coriander haters!

Preparation method: Wash and rinse dry the coriander. Cut off the roots and chop the coriander leaves. Finely chop the ginger slices. Heat up 1 tablespoon of oil over medium heat and sauté the chopped ginger until golden brown. Crack the eggs. Add the sesame oil, white pepper powder, salt, cooked ginger and chopped coriander. Beat the egg mixture. Heat up 1 teaspoon of oil and pour in the beaten egg mixture. Stir the mixture with chopstick and cook for 1 minute or until the bottom turns brown. Flip the omelette and cook for another 30 seconds. Garnish the egg with more coriander leaves on top and serve warm.

9.2 Diaphoretics with Pungent Cool Properties (辛凉解表药)

These diaphoretics are used to treat external wind heat syndrome whose symptoms are fever, body aches, sore throat, thirst, thick mucus with a yellow tinge, cough, red tongue with thin yellow fur, and a floating fast pulse.

(i) Mint (*bohe* 薄荷)

Mint is identified by its light and refreshing smell liked by most people as it makes them feel more alert and uplifts their mood. Mint is believed to originate from Europe and the Mediterranean area, but the best mint arguably comes from Suzhou. The mint used in

Chinese medicine comes in a wide variety which includes peppermint. The leaves and stems have similar medicinal value.

Therapeutic actions: Mint works very well in expelling wind heat pathogens from the head, especially the eyes, nose and throat. Its cool minty nature and uplifting pungent flavour are very effective in clearing nasal congestion and soothing the eyes and throat. Because of the volatile nature of its components, it is best to use fresh mint leaves. One can relieve symptoms by smelling the leaves or crushing them and rubbing onto the temples. Mint also helps to regulate the liver qi, hence it can be used to treat mild depressive moods with chest tightness.

Recipe: Mint and toufu soup 薄荷豆腐汤

Ingredients: 7–8 fresh mint leaves, half a piece toufu, sliced lean pork, spring onions

This cooling soup is ideal for summer with humid weather as mint and tofu are cool and help to relieve summer heat. It is good for the prevention of colds and flu in the summer season. In addition, mint enhances the sympathetic nervous system. Its strong fragrance clears the head and makes one feel less lethargic. Individuals with weak stomachs should not take this soup too often.

Preparation method: Cook the toufu in a pot of boiling water. Add sliced lean pork. Once the lean pork is cooked, add the fresh mint leaves and spring onions and turn off the heat. Add salt to taste and serve warm. Do take note to turn off the fire once the fresh mint leaves are added so that its fragrance is not evaporated by the heat.

(ii) Mulberry leaf (*sangye* 桑叶)
The mulberry tree, the nutritious food source for silkworms, is also filled with goodness for humans. All its parts, including the twig, fruit, and bark have health benefits, with each targeting a different syndrome, with therapeutic actions for the lung and liver.

Therapeutic actions: Mulberry leaf expels wind heat pathogens, clears lung heat and moistens the lung. It is a versatile herb for cough arising from external wind heat syndromes as well as dryness of lung, which presents as a dry cough with little phlegm. It is best used in the initial phase of cough. Mulberry leaf also suppresses the hyperactivity of liver yang and clears liver heat, manifested in headache, dizziness, irritability, and red teary eyes. Fresh mulberry leaf is better at expelling wind heat pathogens than dried leaf. The latter is better in suppressing liver yang, although they can be used interchangeably.

Recipe: Mulberry leaf millet porridge 桑叶小米粥

Ingredients: 6g of dried mulberry leaves, 75g of millet, 2 red dates with seeds removed.

Porridge is one dish that is recommended when one is unwell as it does not damage healthy qi. This recipe is designed for individuals with a weak stomach who have mild cough with constipation. Millet is a good source of fibre. It can help to move the bowels, a problem faced by people who have cough due to poor descending of qi. The cool nature of the mulberry leaf is mitigated by millet and red dates which nourish the spleen and stomach.

Preparation method: Boil the mulberry leaves in water for about 15 to 20 minutes. Remove the mulberry leaves and use the water to cook the millet. Add the red dates and continue to cook for about 20 to 30 minutes. Serve warm.

(iii) Chrysanthemum flower (*juhua* 菊花)

Chrysanthemum flower is one of the most common herbs and widely available from Chinese medical stores. During the Tang dynasty, chrysanthemum flowers were not so easily available and were regarded as one of the precious herbs presented to the emperor. The best quality chrysanthemums are from *Jiaozuo* (焦作) in Henan province where soil, water and climate are optimal for its cultivation. Chrysanthemums grown here, known as *huai juhua* (怀菊花), reputedly have the strongest therapeutic effects.

Therapeutic actions: Chrysanthemum flower and mulberry leaf have similar therapeutic actions and they are often used together. They are a classic example of herb compatibility with mutual reinforcement. Compared mulberry leaf, chrysanthemum flower is weaker in expelling wind heat pathogens and clearing lung heat, but stronger in suppressing liver yang and clearing liver fire. Clinical research suggests that hyperactivity of liver yang is one of the common syndromes in high blood pressure. Hence, suppressing liver yang can help control mild high blood pressure. However, without medical advice, these two herbs should not be used in place of hypertension drugs.

Chrysanthemum flower also has a detoxification action which mulberry leaf does not have. It can be used to treat acute stages of carbuncles, sores and ulcers by removing heat and toxins, thereby reducing swelling.

Recipe: Chrysanthemum tea for promoting vision 菊花明目茶

Ingredients: 9g chrysanthemum flowers, 9g mulberry leaves, 3g wolfberry seeds

This tea is suitable for individuals who have dry, red or teary eyes due to exuberance of liver fire. Chrysanthemum flowers and mulberry leaves clear liver fire and wolfberry seeds nourish liver yin to moisturise the eyes. As this tea is quite cooling, it is not suited to those with weak spleen and stomach.

Preparation method: Wash and rinse the herbs and put the chrysanthemum flowers and mulberry leaves in a pot of water. After the water is boiled, cook the herbs over low heat for about 15 to 20 minutes. During the last 5 minutes, add in the wolfberry seeds. Serve warm.

(iv) Kudzuvine root (*gegen* 葛根)

Kudzuvine root is often mistaken for arrowroot and cassava because of their similar appearances. Kudzuvine root, commonly known as *fenge* (粉葛), is available fresh in the wet markets and is a common ingredient for soups. During famines in China in the past, kudzuvine root was regarded as the main food source because of its high nutritional value and low cost, hence it is also known as Asian ginseng. There are two forms of kudzuvine root: the powdered kudzuvine root (粉葛根) which is used as food because of its high starch content, and the fibrous kudzuvine root (柴葛根) which is used mainly for medicinal purposes.

Therapeutic actions: Kudzuvine root is good for its antipyrectic effect, helping to bring down fever. It can also promote the production of fluids to quench thirst and is effective in alleviating a stiff neck. Therefore, it is a suitable herb to use when treating external wind heat syndrome with fever, thirst, body aches and stiff neck. Its clinical application is not limited to external wind heat syndromes, as it can also relieve thirst arising from internal heat or yin deficiency syndromes. Another use is for relieving diarrhea caused by heat or weakness of spleen and stomach, a therapeutic action that is further enhanced by its capability to uplift yang qi.

    Recent biomedical research suggests that kudzuvine root has vasodilating properties, hence making it a helpful herb for lowering blood pressure and alleviating coronary heart disease.[15] In addition, it contains active ingredients such as puerarin, an isoflavonoid, that has the effect of lowering blood glucose and cholesterol levels.

Recipe: Kudzuvine root with burdock soup 粉葛牛蒡汤

Ingredients: 150g of burdock root (牛蒡), 300g of kudzuvine root, 150g of carrot, 250g of corn, 2 pieces of candied red dates, 2 litres of water, salt

---

[15] Minyan Huang *et al* (2021)

This soup is good for removing heat and toxins, yet not too cooling for someone with a weak stomach. Burdock root is added to enhance the effects of removing heat and toxins. Carrot, corn and red dates are all neutral in nature and nourish the stomach, hence they protect it from the cool nature of kudzuvine and burdock. In addition, carrot has also some mild effect in removing toxins and heat, and corn a diuretic effect, removing excess heat through urination. This is an ideal soup to drink when one is down with a fever from wind heat pathogens and suffers from poor appetite. It can also be consumed on a hot summer day even if one is feeling well!

Preparation method: Peel off the skin of the kudzuvine root and cut into thin slices or small cubes. Peel off the skin of the carrot and burdock and cut them into small pieces. Cut the corn into small pieces too. Pour all ingredients into a pot of water. Add the candied red dates. Cover the pot and boil. Once the water has boiled, lower to medium heat and continue to cook for 1 hour. Add salt to taste and serve warm.

Chapter 10

Herbs and Recipes for Heat, Dampness, Wind and other Internal Conditions

10.1 Heat Clearing Herbs (清热药)

These herbs from medical halls are used to brew the bitter-tasting tea that people drink when they feel "heaty". The main therapeutic action of these herbs is to remove any form of internal heat in the organs, qi and blood. Internal heat can be organ fire such as liver fire, or heat dampness, deficiency heat, or heat associated with toxins. As you may have guessed, most of the heat clearing herbs are either cool or cold in nature.

These herbs should not be consumed for a prolonged period especially for those who have a weak spleen. The cold nature of these herbs can damage spleen qi and yang, causing loose stools, aversion to cold foods and drinks, poor appetite and abdominal pain. One should stop taking heat clearing herbs when internal heat syndrome is resolved.

In clinical practice, heat clearing herbs are often the first choice for treating inflammatory conditions associated with infections. From a biomedical perspective, most heat clearing herbs have anti-bacterial and anti-viral properties which explains why they can be effective for treating inflammatory and infectious diseases. In 2002 during the SARS epidemic and the more recent Covid-19 pandemic, China used heat clearing herbs such as honeysuckle flowers and isatis roots among the main ingredients for treating these diseases. There have been favourable reports of their efficacy.

Some of the main heat clearing herbs used in Chinese medicine are covered below.

(i) Honeysuckle flower (*jinyinhua* 金银花)

Most of us are familiar with the dried form of honeysuckle flower as small green plain-looking buds. The fresh flower, on the other hand, are white when in full bloom, then changes to yellow one or two days later, giving the flower its Chinese name of *jin* (金 gold) *yin* (银 silver) *hua*. Two different colours of flowers can thus be seen on the same plant. *Jinyinhua* (金银花) is also known as the 'lovebirds vine' (*yuanyangteng* 鸳鸯藤) because the gold and silver flowers are always seen together.

Honeysuckle flower grows new sprouts at the end of autumn and continues to grow in winter, as if it was arming itself with winter cold to fight the nasty summer heat to follow. Hence another name for this flower is *rendonghua* (忍冬花) - the flower that withstands winter.

Therapeutic actions: Honeysuckle flower can eliminate both external and internal heat. Hence it can be used for the common cold or flu associated with wind heat external syndromes as well as ulcers, sores, acnes, carbuncles and inflammation of the lung, heart and gastrointestinal caused by internal heat toxin syndromes.

Because of its effectiveness in clearing heat and toxins, the honeysuckle flower is also commonly used to treat infectious diseases such as chicken pox, hand foot mouth diseases and, more recently, Covid-19. Viruses are a form of heat toxin pathogens in TCM. The honeysuckle flower is one of the principal herbs used in *Lianhua Qingwen* (连花清瘟) which is a TCM medication for alleviating early symptoms of Covid-19.

Recipe: *Honeysuckle flower tea* 金银花茶

Ingredients: 5g weeping forsythia (*lianqiao* 连翘), 3g honeysuckle flowers, 3g chrysanthemum flowers

This tea is formulated for individuals with acne accompanied by irritability, body warmness and a red tongue. Honeysuckle flower and weeping forsythia are often used as a pair for heat clearing and detoxification. Chrysanthemum flowers also clear heat. As all three herbs are cool in nature, the tea should not be taken long term or regularly. For acne, it should be taken when the acnes are slightly red, inflamed and painful.

Preparation method: Mash weeping forsythia and honeysuckle flower together. Mix in chrysanthemum and add 300ml of hot water. Infuse the herbs in hot water for 3 to 5 minutes and serve warm. There can be four to five infusions from the same herbs.

(ii) Common selfheal fruit-spike (*xiakucao* 夏枯草)

Originating from Europe, the medicinal properties of this herb have been widely used by the Western herbalists for its wound healing and haemostatic (blood-clotting) effects, which could be the reason for the word 'selfheal' to be in its name. These fruit spikes are also grown in China and harvested in summer when their medicinal value is the strongest.

Therapeutic actions: This herb is commonly known as the "liver herb" as its actions target the liver, mainly purging liver fire. Compared to chrysanthemum flowers and mulberry leaves, it is more effective for clearing liver heat, hence is used to treat sore eyes and headache due to exuberance of liver fire.

This herb disperses abnormal mass or growth to reduce swelling and can be used for scrofula, abscesses, inflammation of the neck lymph nodes and enlargement of the thyroid gland due to liver fire.

Recipe: Cooling tea for clearing liver fire 夏桑菊涼茶

Ingredients: 10g common selfheal fruit-spike, 8g mulberry leaves, 5g chrysanthemum flowers, 1g liquorice root

This formulation is similar to the herbal drink *xiasangju* (夏桑菊) found in medical halls. It comes in powder form or as ready-to-drink tea bags, usually sweetened with sugar to lessen its bitterness.

The tea recipe that we introduce here has liquorice root added to enhance heat clearing and detoxification and to harmonize the combined effects of the herbs. Liquorice also adds sweetness to the tea. This tea is for therapeutic purpose and should not be drunk when one is feeling well.

Preparation method: Rinse all the herbs and add them into a pot of 2 litres of water. Bring the water to boil, then lower heat and continue to cook for another 10 minutes. Serve warm.

(iii) Isatis root (*banlangen* 板蓝根)

This is a short plant with large green leaves which are used for making indigo dye. The root of the plant is used for medicinal purposes.

Therapeutic actions: In China, the isatis root is well known for heat clearing and detoxification and has been widely used in the treatment of infectious diseases such as plaque, mumps, scarlet fever, tonsilitis, influenza, SARS and Covid-19.

It is especially effective for treating sore throat due to heat toxins manifested in a red, painful and swollen throat with or without fever, a red tongue and a fast pulse. A few boxes of isatis root granules or powder at home would be handy for sore throats.

Recipe: *Isatis root tea* 板蓝根茶

Ingredients: 15g honeysuckle flowers, 10g isatis root, 7 pieces of fig

This cooling and mildly sweet flavoured herbal tea is for alleviating sore throat in its early stage, especially when one is having a common cold or flu. Honeysuckle flower clears heat and toxins, and expels external wind heat pathogens. Fig is a sweet fruit that enhances the heat clearing and detoxification actions to reduce swelling, and also promotes the production of fluids to moisturise the throat.

Preparation method: Rinse all the herbs and add them to a pot of 200ml of water. Bring the water to boil, then lower heat and continue to cook for another 10 to 15 minutes. Serve warm.

(iv) Dandelion (*pugongying* 蒲公英)

Dandelion as a food and medicinal herb has been recorded for thousands over of years in Asia as well as ancient Egypt, Greece and Rome. The entire dandelion plant from the flower to the root has medicinal value.

Therapeutic actions: As a herb with heat clearing and detoxification capabilities, dandelion can be used to treat a wide range of inflammatory diseases and infections such as chronic gastritis, sore throat, tonsilitis, dermatitis, and bronchitis. All of these conditions must have the same underlying heat toxin syndrome.

Dandelion is also used in mastitis, an inflammation of milk ducts. This condition is seen in breastfeeding women when they experience painful, lumpy and warm breasts with fever and/or pus forming in the breast. In addition, it can be used to treat carbuncles, boils and furuncles because of its ability to disperse masses to reduce swelling.

Dandelion is also a diuretic and provides a channel to clear heat and toxins through urination. It can also be used in urinary tract infections and jaundice due to heat dampness in the liver.

Recipe: Cold-dish dandelion 凉拌蒲公英

Ingredients: 150g fresh dandelion, 4 cloves of minced garlic, 1 to 2 tablespoons oil, 2 teaspoons black vinegar, 2 teaspoons light soy sauce, sugar and salt to taste. Optional: 1 to 2 shredded dried chilli

This is a simple and appetizing cold dish to release heat. Together with the sauce, this refreshing and cooling dish that comes with a tinge of bitterness helps reduce mild infections. If you are well and do not have a weak and cold spleen, this dish can be eaten as a prophylactic forming part of a meal. Garlic, chilli and black vinegar can be added to mitigate the coolness of the dish.

Preparation method: Blanch the fresh dandelion in salted boiling water for about 10 seconds. Put the blanched dandelion in a bowl of ice water and dry it by squeezing out the water. Place the dandelion on a plate and pour soy sauce, black vinegar, sugar, salt, minced garlic and shredded chilli over it. Heat the oil and pour it over the dandelion.

(v) Indian trumpet flower seed (*muhudie* 木蝴蝶)

The Indian trumpet flower tree is a tall tree with a height of 7.5 to 12 meters. Its seeds are used as medicine. After the fruits are harvested in fall and winter, they are placed under the sun until they are cracked to remove the seeds which are further sunned. The seed resembles a butterfly hence the name 木蝴蝶 (wooden butterfly). It is also known as *qianchenzhi* (千层纸 thousand layered paper).

Therapeutic actions: It is used for its lung heat clearing and throat soothing effects. It also regulates liver qi flow and soothes the stomach. Among the heat clearing herbs mentioned in this chapter, the Indian trumpet flower seed is the least cooling, hence it is suitable for individuals with a weak spleen but experience mild sore throat as a consequence of lung heat. The sore throat is presented as a dry, raspy and slightly painful throat with a hoarse voice. This herb also resolves bloating pain in the side of the ribs and abdominal areas due to liver qi stagnation.

Recipe: *The fire-fighting tea* 清热降火茶

Ingredients: 5g chrysanthemum flowers, 3g honeysuckle flowers, 2g Indian trumpet flower seeds, 3g red dates

This tea is ideal for a slightly painful throat with a hoarse voice and a feeling of heat simmering inside. The three heat clearing herbs douse the fire and soothe the throat without hurting the spleen and stomach. Red dates help to protect the spleen and stomach from the cool nature of the other herbs and also sweeten the tea.

Preparation method: Boil red dates in water for about 15 minutes. Use the water to steep the herbs for 10 to 15 minutes. Serve warm.

(vi) Oldenlandia diffusa (*baihua sheshecao* 白花蛇舌草)
This herb grows in East and Southeast Asia including Singapore. It is a short plant with small white flowers and leaves that resembles a snake's tongue, hence is called snake-needle grass, and in Chinese the "white flower snake tongue grass".

Therapeutic actions: Oldenlandia is a very cool herb with strong heat clearing and detoxification actions. It is known for being anti-inflammatory and believed to have anti-cancer properties. It is effective in reducing swelling and inflammation of boils, carbuncles, and wounds from snake bites via either oral or external application.
Oldenlandia is also able to remove dampness through urination, hence it is used to treat urinary tract infections and jaundice resulting from heat dampness.

Recipe: *Oldenlandia soup with Chinese barley* 苡米白花蛇舌草汤

Ingredients: 60g fresh oldenlandia, 30g Chinese barley, 6g candied melon

This recipe is suitable for individuals who have mild urinary tract infection with heat dampness as the underlying syndrome. Chinese barley promotes urination, enhancing oldenlandia's clearing of heat and resolving dampness. This soup's bitterness is mitigated by candied melon, which also has a diuretic effect.

Preparation method: Rinse the Chinese barley and cook it in a pot of water over low heat for about 1 hour. Rinse the oldenlandia and add to the pot. Continue to cook for 30 minutes. Decant and add candied melon.

(vii) Green bean / Mung bean (*lüdou* 绿豆)
Green bean soup is a popular dessert on a hot day because of its summer heat clearing effect.

Therapeutic actions: Besides clearing summer heat and preventing heat stroke, green beans eliminate toxins and excess water through urination. As such, it can also be used to treat water retention and urination difficulty as well as carbuncles and ulcers especially if these are due to heat toxins.

Green bean is an antidote for toxic herbs such as arsenic and aconite.

Recipe: Green bean soup 绿豆汤

Ingredients: Green beans

Everyone has their own green bean soup recipes with different variations such as adding Chinese barley or sweet potatoes and dried tangerine peel. This basic recipe retains most of the therapeutic benefits of green beans as it is not cooked for hours or sweetened with sugar. Each part of the green bean has a different property: the skin of the green bean is cooling whereas the flesh is neutral. Therefore, it is best to drink the green bean water as well for the full effect of clearing summer heat.

Preparation method: Soak the green beans in water for 10 minutes. Bring it to boil and continue to cook over low heat for 10 minutes. Serve warm.

10.2 Herbs for Resolving Dampness (化湿药)

Dampness is a troublesome pathogen that is hard to eliminate because of its sticky nature. The spleen is often its first victim, hence dampness tends to produce symptoms associated with the poor functioning of the spleen such as bloating, nausea and poor digestion.

Most of the herbs that resolve dampness are attributable to the spleen meridian, and are warm and pungent (辛) so that they have a drying effect on dampness. Taken in excess or for too long, they may cause dryness in the mouth or throat. Not many dampness resolving herbs can be incorporated into medicated foods because of their unpleasant taste. We shall introduce one herb in this category.

White cardamom fruit (*baidoukou* 白豆蔻)

This round, white coloured cardamom fruit is different from the green spindle shaped cardamom that Indians use as a spice although both come from the same family as ginger. The smell and taste of the cardamom fruit are similar to that of ginger but there is a mild peppery taste that uplifts food with its aroma. Being the less popular fruit among the two species, the white cardamom fruit, which originates from Thailand and Cambodia, is widely used as a food ingredient in East Asia, especially China.

Therapeutic actions: *Baidoukou* is warm in nature with a pungent flavour that warms the spleen and resolves dampness that causes qi stagnation manifested in a bloated abdomen, nausea, and poor appetite. *Baidoukou* promotes qi flow and relieves vomiting. It should not be cooked for too long if it is to retain its aroma and therapeutic effects.

Recipe: *Chicken wings simmered with white cardamom fruit* 白豆蔻煨鸡翅

Ingredients: 10 chicken wings (make 2 slits at the back of the chicken wing), 3g white cardamom fruit (soaked in warm water), some ginger and onion slices, green and red capsicums, rice wine, salt and sugar

Most meat dishes tend to make one feel full easily but not with this chicken wings recipe which boosts appetite and relieves a bloated stomach. Ginger and onion are added to enhance qi regulation, which helps digestion of food. Capsicums are warm and resolve dampness. Chicken is chosen because it is a mild spleen qi tonic. This recipe suits a person with a weak and cold spleen and stomach and suffers from a bloated abdomen with poor appetite.

However, this dish is warm and drying, hence it does not suit those with yin deficiency or heat dampness, who might develop constipation and dryness in the mouth or throat.

Preparation method: Preheat the wok. Without adding oil, place the side of the chicken wings with the two slits on the wok. Add rice wine and pan fry the wings over low heat. Flip the wings to prevent them from sticking onto the wok. Once one side of the wing has turned brown, add ginger and onion slices. Stir fry until fragrant. Add soy sauce and water gradually. Add the cardamom fruit together with the water in which it is soaked. Add salt and sugar to taste. Without covering the wok, simmer the chicken wings for about 12 minutes. Remove the ginger and onion. Add the capsicums and corn starch and serve warm.

10.3 Diuretics (利尿药)

If you are urinating more frequently after a meal, it may be that one of the ingredients in your meal has a diuretic effect. In TCM, diuretics are a category of herbs that promotes urination to remove internal pathogens like heat, dampness, phlegm or excess water. Most diuretics are neutral and bland, and are suitable for most body constitutions. Among the common clinical disorders that need diuretics are urinary tract infections and edema (water retention).

(i) Poria (*fuling* 茯苓)

Wild poria is a yam-like fungus that grows underground beneath dead pine trees. It feeds on the nutrients of the pine tree roots and can weigh up to 1.2kg. The use of poria as a food dates back to the Song dynasty. In the late Qing dynasty, poria was made into poria cake (茯苓饼) by imperial physicians to improve the health of Empress dowager *Cixi*. Even to today, traditional poria cake is widely sold as a sweet snack in China.

Therapeutic actions: Poria is suitable for most people because of its neutral and bland properties. It helps to drain dampness and excess water through urination and has a mild qi-invigorating effect on the spleen. It is also helpful in alleviating diarrhea due to a weak spleen, and is used in the formulation *Sishentang* (四神汤). Poria tranquilises the mind to improve sleep and is suitable for those with insomnia with heart palpitation and anxiety due to qi and blood deficiency of the spleen and heart.

Recipe: *Poria milk* 茯苓奶

Ingredients: 500g milk, 10g poria powder, honey (optional)

Poria milk helps people with spleen and stomach deficiency and insomnia. This beverage was believed to be Emperor Qianlong's favourite drink every night before bed. Milk nourishes blood and calms the heart for sleep.

Preparation method: Add poria powder into 100g of milk and keep stirring to dissolve the powder. Put the pot onto the stove. Add the remaining milk and keep stirring until boiling. After the milk has boiled, simmer the milk over low heat for about two to three minutes. Add a few teaspoons of honey to help the powder dissolve better.

(ii) Job's Tears (*yiyiren* 薏苡仁)

Job's tears, also known as Chinese barley, is native to Southeast Asia and later introduced to China and India. The name is derived from the shiny tear shaped husk. There are two varieties of Job's tears. The cultivated variety is used in medicine and cooking because of its soft shell, whereas wild Job's tears have harder shells and are used as ornamental beads.

Therapeutic actions: Job's tears is a cool diuretic which drains dampness and excess water, and also clears heat. It is suitable for treating heat dampness with symptoms of thick greasy yellow coating on the tongue. It is useful for urinary tract infections and poor flow of urine with painful and burning sensation, joint pain with red swelling, and discharging pus of carbuncles and abscesses. Its spleen invigorating effect is enhanced when it is processed by stir frying, which makes it warmer and better for treating diarrhea and water retention.

Job's tears should not be used in pregnant women especially in the first trimester when pregnancy may be less stable. A safer period is the third trimester when the pregnancy is stable, during which it can be used to relieve water retention.

Recipe: Mushroom Job's tears porridge 香菇薏苡仁粥

Ingredients: 100g rice (soaked for 30 minutes), 80g stir-fried Job's tears (soaked for 2 hours), 20g mushrooms (diced), 10g prawn skin, 100ml to 150ml chicken or vegetable stock

This is a piping hot nourishing porridge for those with weakened spleen and heat dampness with typical symptoms of bloated abdomen, poor appetite, loose and sticky stools or diarrhea, sluggishness, mild water retention, pale red tongue with slight teeth indentations and greasy yellow coating. Cooking Job's tears with rice helps to soften the overall texture of the porridge. Mushroom nourishes the stomach and prawn skin regulates qi which in turn boosts appetite. This recipe is not suitable for pregnant women.

Preparation method: Add the soaked rice and Job's tears, together with the water in which it is soaked to the pot. Add more water and cook for 30 minutes. Stir fry the mushrooms, add prawn skin and continue to stir fry until fragrant. Pour the stock into the pot and add stir-fried mushrooms and prawn skin. Continue to cook until the porridge is boiling. Serve warm.

(iii) Winter melon skin (*dongguapi* 冬瓜皮)

Ironically, winter melon grows in summer and is harvested in autumn, not winter. Its name derives from the frosty look of the skin of the ripened fruit. Most people remove the skin of winter melon during cooking but may not realise they have discarded the valuable cooling part of the fruit.

Therapeutic actions: The skin of the winter melon promotes urination and is commonly used to relieve water retention by pairing it with different herbs. As the skin is difficult to chew and digest, only the water from cooking the skin is normally used. If water retention is due to a cold syndrome with symptoms such as swollen eyelids in the morning, aversion to cold, fatigue, less urine output and soft stools, a drink of winter melon skin and ginger (a warm herb) may resolve the problem. If it is a heat syndrome with a feeling of warmth, thirst, scanty urine and constipation, cook winter melon skin with red bean (a cool herb). Winter melon skin promotes lactation and can be added to fish soups. Both the fresh and dried forms winter melon skin have medicinal value, although the dried ones are the preferred as they are more concentrated.

Recipe: *Winter melon soup with Job's tears*

Ingredients: 500g winter melon with the skin, 50g Job's tears, 150g pork ribs, 3g dried tangerine peel

This soup kills two birds with one stone: it reduces water retention and also helps with weight loss. As both winter melon skin and Job's tears are cooling, a small amount of warm-natured dried tangerine peel is added to warm the soup a bit. Those with qi and yang deficiency in the spleen and stomach should not drink this soup.

Preparation method: Fill the pot with water. Add winter melon, Job's tears and pork ribs. Bring to boil and cook over low heat for 2 hours. Add dried tangerine peel 30 minutes before serving. Season with salt and serve warm.

(iv) Corn silk (*yumixu* 玉米须)

Corn silk is the shiny thread-like silky fibres that protrude from the tip of the ear of corn, hence the name 'dragon's whiskers' (龙须)

or 'pearls on the crown' (皇冠上的珍珠). Like winter melon skin, corn silk is often discarded during cooking by those who do not know its medicinal benefits.

Therapeutic actions: Corn silk is a sweet and neutral food that promotes diuresis to relieve water retention and remove jaundice. In China, corn silk is used in the treatment of nephrology conditions as some studies suggest that it can reduce protein in urine.

If fresh corn silk is used, a larger dose of 60g to 120g is required to achieve the desired therapeutic effects. Generally, it is suitable for most body constitutions.

Recipe: *Corn silk tea with dendrobium* 玉米须石斛茶

Ingredients: 30g dried corn silk or 60g fresh corn silk, 6g dendrobium

A simple tea that promotes urination and nourishes yin, hence it is suited for individuals who are experiencing less urine output with thirst and dry mouth.

Preparation method: Either infuse the herbs in hot water for 10 minutes or boil them for 20 minutes for a more concentrated tea.

10.4 Interior Warming Herbs (温里药)

Interior warming herbs are used to resolve internal cold, an excess syndrome, and can also help with yang deficiency. They have a strong pungent flavour to dispel the cold pathogens which tend to attack the spleen and kidney. Most of these herbs are available from supermarkets as they are ordinary spices that we use in cooking. As with diaphoretics, these herbs should not be cooked for too long in order that they retain their pungent flavour.

(i) Dried ginger (*ganjiang* 干姜)
There is this old saying 'The older the ginger, the spicier it is' (姜还是老的辣). Besides acknowledging experience in life and in work, the saying does have a medical basis in that old ginger is warmer

with a more intense pungency. Dried ginger is made by drying the old ginger in the sun, changing the nature of the old ginger from warm to hot.

Therapeutic actions: While fresh ginger resolves external cold syndromes, dried ginger is hotter and stronger for dispelling cold pathogens from the spleen and stomach. It is used to treat internal cold syndrome and spleen yang deficiency manifested in gastric pain, bloating, vomiting and loose stools or diarrhoea that worsens after taking cold foods.

Dried ginger is also used in the treatment of cough and dyspnea (laboured breathing) due to cold rheum with clear runny phlegm. Breathing steam from water with boiled dried ginger is a home remedy for dispelling the cold pathogens from the lung.

Recipe: *Dried ginger red tea with liquorice root* 干姜甘草红茶

Ingredients: 5g dried ginger, 5g honey-baked liquorice root, 7g red tea leaves

This tea helps to alleviate stomach discomfort or pain especially after taking food or drinks of cold nature. It is also suitable for individuals who have spleen yang deficiency. Red tea is chosen because of its warmth. Honey-baked liquorice root nourishes the spleen and stomach, and its sweetness mitigates the pungent flavour of dried ginger. This tea is not suitable for those with a heaty body constitution.

Preparation method: Cut the dried ginger and liquorice root into thin slices. Infuse all ingredients in hot water for 5 to 10 minutes.

(ii) Cassia bark (*rougui* 肉桂)

Cassia bark or Chinese cinnamon originates from Guangxi, China. It is different from the spice used in cooking known as Ceylon cinnamon, or *guipi* (桂皮), which is darker, thinner and more fragrant, and has weaker medicinal properties. Cassia bark is used mainly for medicinal purposes. It is extremely hot and prescribed in low doses as it contains coumarin which is toxic if taken in excess.

Therapeutic actions: Cassia bark is used for severe kidney yang deficiency. Its effect is similar to that of antler's horn. It also dispels internal cold pathogens and warms the collaterals to relieve pain. As such, it is used to treat infertility, menstrual disorders, and abdominal and back pain resulting from kidney yang deficiency or internal cold syndromes.

To warm the kidney, one teaspoon of cassia bark powder mixed into yellow wine and made into a paste can be placed on the acupoint *yongquan* (涌泉) at the base of the feet.

Because cassia bark is very hot, it may not be suitable for pregnant women.

Recipe: Cassia bark tea with honey 蜂蜜肉桂茶

Ingredients: ½ to 1 teaspoon cassia bark powder, 2 teaspoon honey

This tea warms the body and may be drunk before breakfast or sleep. Drinking it on an empty stomach ensures that the tea is well absorbed to start the day with a boost of yang qi. Before sleep, it calms the mind. Honey nourishes spleen qi and softens the pungency of the cassia bark.

Preparation method: Add cassia bark powder into hot water. Add honey after it has cooled down a bit.

(iii) Fennel seed (*xiaohuixiang* 小茴香)

Highly aromatic although milder than star anise, the fennel seed is one of the ingredients in "five spices powder" used in Chinese cooking. It comes from a flowering plant in the carrot family, indigenous to the Mediterranean. The seed has higher medicinal value than other parts of the plant because of its high essential oil content.

Therapeutic actions: Unlike dried ginger and cassia bark which can restore yang, the fennel seed is better for dispelling cold pathogens and regulating qi to relieve pain. It is used in such conditions as abdominal pain, menstrual pain, testicle pain, bloating, and poor appetite due to cold pathogens in the organs.

There is no recipe for this herb as it is commonly used as a spice in many dishes. However, as this herb has a very strong flavour and may cause dryness in the throat and mouth, it is recommended to use this versatile ingredient in smaller amounts.

(iv) Clove (*dingxiang* 丁香)
Clove is the flower bud of the tree of the Myrtaceae family. In ancient times, cloves were not easily available to the commoners in China. Its fragrance made it popular as a breath freshener, presentable as a gift to the imperial family.

Therapeutic actions: In addition to dispelling cold pathogens, clove also warms the abdomen and promotes the descent of stomach qi to relieve vomiting, burping, diarrhea and abdominal discomfort from the cold pathogens in the stomach. It also warms the kidney to strengthen yang and can help with male impotency.

Used as a spice to reduce the smell of the meat, clove improves digestion of the meal. Like fennel seeds, it should be used only in small amounts.

Recipe: Clove patch for relieving diarrhea 丁香止泻贴

Ingredients: 3g clove, 3g cassia bark, yellow wine

This is an external application for relieving diarrhea caused by yang deficiency in the spleen and kidney with symptoms of loose or watery stools especially near dawn, aversion to cold, nausea, vomiting and abdominal pain that is relieved by warm compression. It may be used for children. Clove and cassia bark are used together for warming the spleen and kidney. It is advisable not to take foods that are cold and hard to digest when using this patch.

Preparation method: Grind both herbs into powder. Add sufficient yellow wine to mix them into a paste and put it on a white gauze. Place it on the navel, acupoints *zusanli* (足三里) or *zhongwan*

(中脘) for 1 hour. The duration of use can increase slowly to 24 hours depending on the condition.

(v) Pepper (*hujiao* 胡椒)

Black and white pepper come from the same flowering vine. Black pepper is the unripe drupe of the pepper plant while white pepper comes from the seed of the ripened fruit. White pepper is hotter and more pungent than black pepper, although they share the same actions.

Therapeutic actions: As pepper warms the stomach and dispels cold pathogens, most people are comfortable eating it. It promotes the descent of qi and resolves phlegm. Besides alleviating abdominal pain, diarrhoea and vomiting caused by internal cold syndromes, pepper can also be used with other herbs to treat epilepsy due to phlegm. It may also counteract toxins in seafood.

It is recommended to use whole white peppercorn for maximum therapeutic effect. To retain its volatile components, it should not be cooked for too long.

Recipe: *White peppercorn mushroom chicken soup* 白胡椒香菇鸡汤

Ingredients: 6 mushrooms, 3 red dates (seeds removed), 9 slices old ginger, 6 garlic cloves, 400g chicken leg (chop into big pieces), 1 tablespoon white peppercorn, ½ teaspoon salt, sesame oil, Shaoxing wine and wolfberry seeds

This peppery chicken soup is good for cold rainy days, as it neutralizes cold pathogens in the spleen and stomach and nourishes spleen qi. It can be considered a modified version of the classic *bakkuteh* dish (peppery pork rib soup) but uses fewer spices. Old ginger enhances the warming action of white peppercorn; garlic is pungent and regulates the stagnated spleen qi. Chicken is used instead of pork as it is a qi tonic food. Red dates nourish the stomach. Sesame oil and Shaoxing wine enhance the warmness of the soup. This soup is particularly suited to persons who suffer from abdominal pain or bloating from coldness, but not for those who already have internal heat.

Preparation method: Wash the mushrooms and soak them in warm water for at least 40 minutes. Peel off the skin and crush the garlic. Blanch the chicken pieces in a pot of boiling water with 3 slices of old ginger and some Shaoxing wine. Take out the chicken once the water starts to boil again. Pour 1 teaspoon of sesame oil in a clay pot and sauté the white peppercorns and garlic in it. Add 1200ml of water. Add chicken, mushrooms, red dates, the remaining 6 slices of old ginger, 1 tablespoon of Shaoxing wine and 300ml of the mushroom water. Bring to boil and continue to simmer it over low heat for 40 minutes. Turn off the fire and add wolfberry seeds and salt.

(vi) Prickly ash peel (*huajiao* 花椒)

Famous Sichuan spice prickly ash peel is the skin of the ripened fruit of a spiky shrub. It has a numbing effect on the tongue and together with hot pepper give Sichuan cuisine the unique taste of *mala* (麻辣), or hot and numbing. Though not a pepper, it is known as the Sichuan pepper or *shujiao* (蜀椒). During the Western Han dynasty, palace walls of empresses were painted with *huajiao* powder. The appearance of many fruits on a twig in auspicious red colour signified bearing many sons. *Huajiao* also dispels cold and dampness and protected wooden structures from parasites.

Therapeutic actions: Besides dispelling cold pathogens, prickly ash peel removes body dampness via sweating. Sichuan province suffers from high humidity, hence their folks feel comfortable and lighter after a meal with prickly ash peel.

Another special property of prickly ash peel is that it kills parasites like roundworms that cause abdominal pain, and scabies or mites which cause eczema and vaginal itch. Treatment is by boiling the herb and using the water to wash the skin.

Overuse of this herb damages yin, leading to constipation and excessive sweating that exhausts qi.

Recipe: Prickly ash peel foot bath 花椒泡脚水

Ingredients: 20 to 30g prickly ash peel

This foot bath is suitable for fungus infection as prickly ash peel kills parasites. It can also be used to alleviate cold feet and pain in the legs due to cold dampness.

Preparation method: Boil the prickly ash peel in a pot of water for 15 minutes. Cool to a comfortable temperature and soak both feet for 20 to 30 minutes. Soak for 3 consecutive days for better results.

10.5 Herbs for Promoting Digestion (消食药)

This category of herbs aids in the digestion of food and resolves bloating, excessive burping, nausea and poor appetite. These herbs also help with indigestion problems in children.

(i) Hawthorn (*shanzha* 山楂)

Hawthorn is a berry-like fruit of the Crataegus plant, used to make hawthorn cake, also known as the "golden cake" (金糕), served in ancient times to imperial families. Today, hawthorn is used to make sweet snacks such as haw flakes or glazed fruits.

Therapeutic actions: Hawthorn is known for its meat tenderizing effect and was used by the famous poet and culinary expert *Su Dong Po* (苏东波) to stew with chicken. It aids digestion, especially of meat. Hawthorn tea should be taken only after meals as its sourness may irritate the gastric lining or trigger reflux.

Hawthorn also promotes blood flow and relieves menstruation cramps resulting from blood stasis. Biomedical research suggests that hawthorn supports cardiovascular health by lowering lipids and keeping blood vessels elastic.

Pregnant women, especially those who are in their first trimester, should avoid taking hawthorn as its promotion of blood flow may pose a risk to pregnancy.

Recipe: Braised ribs with hawthorn sauce 山楂排骨

Ingredients: 1kg pork ribs (chopped into pieces), 10g dried hawthorn slices, half lemon cut into slices with seeds removed, 2 scallion stalks (cut into short segments), ½ ginger (cut into 8 slices), 6 cloves of garlic (crushed), 15 to 20g rock sugar, 1 tablespoon soy sauce, 1 tablespoon oyster sauce

For the meat lovers, this recipe can reduce the unhealthy effect of fats in the meat and promote its digestion. Lemon enhances the sourness of the dish, making it more appetizing.

Preparation method: Add 1 teaspoon of cooking wine in a pot of hot water and blanch the pork ribs for 5 to 10 minutes. Heat oil in a wok and caramelize the rock sugar with some water. Once the caramelized sugar has turned coffee colour, add 500ml of water. Add all the ingredients except pork ribs. Add soy sauce and oyster sauce and stir. Wash the pork ribs and add to the wok. Cover the wok and simmer over low heat for about 15 minutes. Add lemon slices 8 minutes later. Turn up the heat and continue to stir fry the pork ribs until the sauce is thickened and absorbed. Serve warm.

(ii) Malt (*maiya* 麦芽)

Malt is a partially germinated barley that is made by the malting process in which the grains are soaked in water to germinate for three days and the germination process then halted by sun drying with hot air. During this process, the grains produce enzymes to convert starch into sugar. Malt is a popular ingredient for sweet snacks such as malt sugar (麦芽糖) and dragon's beard candy (龙须糖).

Therapeutic actions: Malt is neutral in nature. It promotes digestion, especially of foods that are high in carbohydrates, regulates qi, strengthens the spleen and improves appetite.

Unprocessed (raw) malt is good for strengthening the spleen and promoting breast milk production, and is suitable for breastfeeding mothers who have spleen qi deficiency with low milk production. Stir-fried malt has stronger action in promoting digestion and regulating qi flow, and is good for relieving indigestion and bloating from overconsumption of starch. Unlike raw malt, it inhibits breast milk production, hence should be used for mothers who wish to wean off breastfeeding. Burnt malt, made by stir frying raw malt to charcoal, is the best for promoting digestion, and is used often in clinical practice.

Recipe: Malt tea 麦芽茶

Ingredients: 10g stir-fried malt, 3g black tea leaves

This is the best choice for a cup of tea to go along with a starchy meal. The combination of stir-fried malt with warm natured black tea warms and nourishes the stomach for good digestion. This tea is suitable for most adults other than pregnant or lactating women.

Preparation method: Put the stir-fried malt into a pot of water and bring it to boil, then simmer for 5 minutes. Use the boiled malt water to infuse the black tea leaves.

(iii) Radish seed (*laifuzi* 莱菔子)

Unlike radish, which is used as food, small reddish brown radish seeds found in the pods of the radish plant are used primarily for medicinal purposes.

Therapeutic actions: Radish and its seeds regulate qi, promote digestion and resolve phlegm. The seeds have stronger pungent flavour hence are better for regulating qi. Among the three digestive herbs covered in this chapter, radish seed is most effective in relieving abdominal bloating from indigestion.

Radish seed resolves phlegm and relieves cough and can be used for both hot and cold syndromes of cough because of its neutral property. It is also commonly used to treat wet cough in the elderly with breathlessness, copious clear phlegm, loss of appetite, bloated stomach and thick white fur. Radish seed is contraindicated for pregnant women as it promotes the descendent of qi which may put the pregnancy at risk. It should not be combined with ginseng as it reduces the medicinal effect of ginseng.

Similar to malt, stir-fried radish seed is gentler on the spleen and stomach, hence it is better for digestion.

Recipe: Porridge with radish seeds 莱菔子粥

Ingredients: 30 to 50g rice, 10 to 15g stir-fried radish seeds

This porridge is suitable for the elderly with chronic cough as well as children with indigestion and poor appetite. Taking the porridge twice a day for two days should bring about some improvement in the condition.

Preparation method: Grind the radish seeds into powder. Wash the rice and cook it into a porridge. Add 5 to 7g of radish seed powder and cook for a while more before serving.

10.6 Herbs for Resolving Phlegm (化痰药)

These herbs resolve phlegm and help relieve cough and dyspnea (breathlessness). They are further classified into herbs for resolving heat phlegm and those for resolving wet phlegm.

(i) Bulb of tendrilleaf fritillary (*chuanbeimu* 川贝母) and Bulb of thunberg fritillary (*zhebeimu* 浙贝母)

Both bulbs come from the same plant genus *Fritillaria*. The bulb of tendrilleaf fritillary (*chuanbeimu*) is more expensive as it is an endangered species that grows only in the wild, mainly in Sichuan. It is used in home remedies for cough. The bulb of thunberg fritillary (*zhebeimu*) is cultivated mostly in Zhejiang province.

Therapeutic actions: The two herbs have similar actions and properties. *Chuanbeimu* is moisturizing and used in chronic cough with scanty sputum and dry throat. The popular Chinese proprietary medicine *Chuanbei pipagao* (川贝枇杷膏) is more suitable for dry cough as its key ingredient is *chuanbeimu*.

Zhebeimu is cooler and more bitter, making it more effective in resolving phlegm and cough. It is used to treat acute chesty cough with viscous yellow or green phlegm.

A common use of both herbs is for reducing swelling by dispersing abnormal mass of phlegm accumulation. *Zhebeimu* has a stronger effect and is often the first choice for treating boils, breast and lung abscesses.

A recipe for this herb is described in the next section on apricot seed.

(ii) Apricot seed (*xingren* 杏仁)

These white coloured heart shaped seeds used in Chinese soups are different from almond nuts. Apricot seed comes from the apricot fruit, and there are two types. The sweet (southern) and bitter (northern) apricot seeds can be used in cooking although the latter contains amygdalin, a toxin that causes cyanide poisoning if taken in excess. Processing and cooking reduces toxicity hence cooked bitter apricot seeds may be consumed in moderate amounts.

Therapeutic actions: As a medicinal herb, the bitter apricot seed is chosen over the sweet apricot seed because it is stronger for resolving phlegm, cough and dyspnea. Its high oil content moistures the large intestine for better bowel movement which is further enhanced by its action of promoting the descent of lung qi. Thus, it is a useful neutral herb for treating cough arising from any syndromes, especially if it is accompanied by constipation.

Recipe: Double boiled snow pear dessert 川贝杏仁炖雪梨

Ingredients: 1 snow pear, preferably with brown skin, 5g *chuanbeimu and zhebeimu* each, 5g bitter apricot seeds, 10g sweet apricot seeds, 3 pieces of candied winter melon

This dessert relieves chronic dry cough with scanty or sticky white sputum as it moisturizes the lung and resolves phlegm. Snow pear with the skin intact enhances lung moisturizing effect and soothes the dry respiratory tract. Candied winter melon is chosen instead of rock sugar as it relieves cough. This recipe should not be used if have thick yellow phlegm as its sweetness may produce more phlegm.

Preparation method: Wash the snow pear and cut it into 4 slices without removing the skin. Rinse the herbs and put them together with the pear in a small clay pot. Add candied winter melon and pour water into the pot to about one third level of the ingredients. Cover the pot and double boil in a pot of water for 1 to 1.5 hours.

(iii) Monk fruit (*luohanguo* 罗汉果)

Luohanguo (monk fruit) comes from Guangxi, China. When ready for harvesting, it changes from green to yellow, after which it is kept in a cool well ventilated place for 7 to 10 days to dry. During this period, the enzymes in the fruit help to convert some carbohydrates into sugar. It is then baked at 80°C to 100°C to a yellowish-brown colour that contains the best therapeutic effects. *Luohanguo* that is dark or black in colour is overbaked.

Therapeutic actions: *Luohanguo* is cool and sweet, clears lung heat, soothes the throat and resolves phlegm, hence is good for relieving warm coughs. Like apricot seeds, it moisturizes the large intestine to promote bowel movement, thus is suitable for cough with constipation due to lung heat syndrome.

There is a newer type of *luohanguo* which is golden in colour and claimed to have better medicinal effect. It is processed using low temperature to vacuum extract moisture from the fruit.

The sweetness of the monk fruit is not a concern to diabetics because it comes from mogrosides produced during processing.

Although it tastes much sweeter than sucrose, it has very few calories and little impact on the blood sugar level.

Recipe: *Monk fruit tea* 罗汉果茶

Ingredient: ½ monk fruit

Processed monk fruit itself is very good for cough. It is important not to remove the skin as it is better than the flesh for moisturizing the lung. A good quality monk fruit is one that is round with no crack, yellowish-brown in colour, and no sound is heard upon shaking the fruit.

Preparation method: Crack the monk fruit with its skin intact and cook it in hot water with a temperature of 80°C to 90°C for 15 minutes.

(iv) Malva seed (*pangdahai* 胖大海)

Malva seed is an essential ingredient of the traditional *cheng teng* (清汤) dessert. It is a seed from the tree species of the Malvaceae family native to Southeast Asia. Besides, Malva seed is also commonly used for culinary purposes in Laos, Vietnam, Cambodia, and Thailand. Although it is a seed, the flesh around it swells to eight times its original size when soaked in water, forming an irregularly shaped, reddish gelatinous mass, hence its Chinese name (胖大海) which means a "fat ocean".

Therapeutic actions: The malva seed has the same actions as the monk fruit although it is weaker in strength. It is frequently used in soups and desserts rather than prescriptions. Malva seed is not toxic but one should not take more than 3 pieces each day as overconsumption can have side effects like white watery phlegm, nausea, coughing, and a swollen tongue. It should be avoided when suffering from diarrhoea.

Recipe: *Malva seed tea* 胖大海茶

Ingredients: 2 pieces of malva seeds, 5g raw liquorice root

This cooling tea suits those who have mild cough with dry throat and hoarse voice, especially cough from throat irritation. Raw liquorice root is added for its heat clearing and detoxification actions, which enhances the soothing of the throat. This tea should be taken after meals to prevent its coolness from damaging the spleen.

Preparation method: Boil the herbs in a pot of water for 10 to 15 minutes. Remove the liquorice root and the core of the malva seed before drinking the tea.

(v) Ginkgo nut (*baiguo* 白果)

Ginkgo nut is the seed found in the fruit of the Ginkgo tree. It is a valuable medical plant with many health benefits. Ginkgo nut is also a popular food ingredient in Asia, for example in the famous ginkgo barley with bean curd dessert.

Therapeutic actions: The ginkgo nut and leaf have similar medicinal properties. Although both relieve coughs, the leaf is valued for its blood flow promoting effect whereas the nut is stronger for relieving cough and dyspnea. Among the herbs for resolving phlegm, ginkgo nut is one of the few that has an astringent flavour, which enables it to relieve cough and dyspnea by astringing the lung, stop abnormal vaginal discharges, and reduce urination. This neutral herb is suitable for most types of coughs except for coughs caused by heat syndrome. It is also used in the treatment of asthma because of its effectiveness in relieving dyspnea.

Ginkgo nut is slightly toxic and should not be taken in excess especially when it is raw. The safest way to consume ginkgo nut is to remove the shell and cook it to facilitate easy removal of the embryo and red membrane that encases the seed, which contains most of the toxins. Cooking reduces the toxicity of ginkgo nut but it does not eliminate it totally. Therefore, one should limit the intake of cooked ginkgo nut to not more than 50 each day. Children, especially 5 years and below, should not eat it as they are more susceptible to acute poisoning which causes convulsion, confusion, nausea, vomiting, abdominal pain and diarrhea 1 to 2 hours after ingestion.

Recipe: Ginkgo nut porridge with bean curd 腐竹白果粥

Ingredients: 220g rice, 30g dried bean curd, 5 litres of water, 50g ginkgo nut, 1g salt, 2g oil, 2 slices ginger

This porridge is ideal for the elderly or individuals who have cough or asthma with spleen and lung qi deficiency. It helps to relieve cough and dyspnea, and also nourishes the spleen to strengthen the body for quick recovery. Bean curd is added to moisturize the lung and resolve phlegm.

Preparation method: Wash and dry the rice. Add salt and oil into the rice and stir. Soak the dried bean curd for at least 20 minutes to soften it. Cut them into smaller pieces and set aside. Remove the shells and cook the ginkgo nuts to remove the membranes and embryos. Once the pot of water has boiled, add all the ingredients. When the water has boiled again, lower the heat and continue to cook for 90 minutes until the texture of the porridge is thick and smooth.

10.7 Herbs for Calming the Liver (平肝药)

Endogenous wind is an internal pathogen that is produced from the hyperactivity of liver yang. It shares similar characteristics as the climatic wind pathogens which includes sudden onset and high mobility. Endogenous wind tends to result in symptoms such as tremors, dizziness and spasms such as are seen in stroke, paralysis, Parkinson's disease and hypertension.

Herbs for calming the liver are attributable to the liver meridian. They calm the liver mainly by extinguishing endogenous wind and suppressing the hyperactivity of liver yang. Most of these herbs are in the form of either minerals or worms, making most of them unsuitable to be used in medicated foods.

Tall gastrodia tuber (*tianma* 天麻)

The tall gastrodia tuber is a perennial herb in the family of Orchidaceae. It is an unusual plant with no leaves and roots but has small resupinate brownish red flowers that resemble red arrows. It is native to Sichuan and Yunnan and is currently under the international protection as an endangered species, which explains its high cost.

Therapeutic actions: As a herb used to resolve hyperactivity of liver yang syndrome, *tianma* treats headaches, dizziness, epilepsy and tremors by suppressing liver yang and extinguishing endogenous wind. It also expels wind and clears the collaterals to relieve arthritic pain and numbness in the limbs especially in stroke patients.

This herb, which is sweet and neutral, is a mild kidney and liver tonic. Long term consumption of it nourishes kidney essence, hence strengthens the knees and back. Recent studies suggest that it dilates the arteries in the brain, hence increasing blood flow to the brain, and may therefore be useful for preventing dementia and insomnia. It may be a suitable herb for patients who have cerebrovascular illnesses such as Alzheimer's disease, Parkinson's disease and stroke. It has been demonstrated that its active ingredients have a tranquilising effect on the mind, hence its possible application for certain mental conditions such as anxiety disorder and depression.

The dried tuber has a stronger therapeutic effect than the fresh one. It should not be over cooked because of the volatility of its active components.

Recipe: Duck stew with tall gastrodia tuber 天麻老鸭煲

Ingredients: Half a duck (chopped into smaller pieces), 10g dried tall gastrodia tuber (soaked for 24 hours), 2 to 3 slices ginger, a small handful of spring onions and wolfberries, salt, rice wine, light soy sauce

This recipe can help alleviate insomnia resulting from anxiety. People who do not sleep well tend to develop liver yin deficiency with deficiency fire. Duck and wolfberries are both yin tonics.

This medicated dish is neutral in nature, making it suitable for most body constitutions.

Preparation method: Chopped soaked tall gastrodia tuber into small pieces. Stir fry the duck in oil. Add ginger and spring onions. Add light soy sauce and rice wine and stir fry until the duck changes colour. Add tall gastrodia tubers and boiled water until it covers the duck. Cook for 30 to 45 minutes. Add salt and wolfberries.

Chapter 11

Herbs and Recipes for Regulating Qi, Promoting Blood Flows, Hemostasis, and Others

11.1 Qi Regulating Herbs (理气药)

To "regulate" qi is to resolve qi stagnation and promote its smooth flow in the body. Qi stagnation symptoms typically are bloatedness, abdominal pain, regurgitation, burping, pain on the sides of the rib cage, depressive moods, and chest tightness. Qi stagnation is often associated with TCM organs like the spleen, stomach, liver and lungs.

Qi regulating herbs are mostly warm and pungent in flavour.

(i) Dried tangerine peel (*chenpi* 陈皮)

Dried tangerine peels (*chenpi*) are the skin of the citrus fruit *Citrus reticulata cv. Chachiensis* (*chazhigan* 茶枝柑). They look similar to the mandarin oranges but have different therapeutic properties. *Chenpi* must be dried and stored for at least 3 years before they are used as medicine. The longer it ages, the stronger its therapeutic action.

Therapeutic actions: *Chenpi* regulates qi and invigorates the spleen. It is used to treat spleen and stomach qi stagnation whose typical symptom is abdominal bloatedness. In most cases of spleen qi stagnation, the main culprit is dampness, which is "sticky" and impairs qi flow. *Chenpi* also dries dampness to restore qi flow and helps to resolve wet phlegm, hence its use for cough due to cold or wet phlegm.

Recipe: Dried tangerine peel with pu'er tea 陈皮普洱茶

Ingredients: 2g dried tangerine peel, 6g pu'er tea leaves

The dried tangerine peel helps with qi stagnation while pu'er aids digestion. This tea is best after a heavy meal.

Preparation method: Put tangerine peel and pu'er tea leaves in a tea pot. Boil water and use it to rinse the tea leaves. Add another 250ml of hot water and infuse for 10 minutes.

(ii) Finger citron (*foshou* 佛手)

Finger citron is a variety of citron whose fruit is made up of finger-like sections. Hence it is also known as Buddha's hand, which in Chinese culture represents happiness and longevity. It has a strong refreshing fragrance which drives its qi regulating action.

Therapeutic actions: Liver qi stagnation is often brought on by emotional stress that impairs the function of the spleen. The finger citron regulates qi and is especially useful for symptoms caused by liver qi stagnation that disturbs spleen and stomach harmony. It helps with pain at the side of the ribs, depressive moods, bloatedness and poor appetite. The finger citron also dries dampness and resolves wet phlegm.

Recipe: Finger citron honey drink

Ingredients: Finger citron and honey

This is a simple fragrant drink to ease bloatedness. Honey is a sweetener but also a mild tonic for spleen and stomach.

Preparation method: Slice the finger citron and dry in the sun. Soak the finger citron in hot water for 2 to 3 minutes, then add honey.

(iii) Rose buds (*meiguihua* 玫瑰花)

Rose used in Chinese medicine is the species *Rosa rugose* native to east Asia and south-eastern Siberia. It grows on beach coasts and sand dunes. Only flower buds that have not bloomed are used as medicine.

Therapeutic actions: Rose buds regulate liver qi and help with depressive moods and menstrual issues (irregular menstruation). It also promotes blood flow therefore is good for gastric pain, breast tenderness, menstrual cramps, trauma and injuries. As it enables better flow of qi and blood, it can enhance facial complexion.

Recipe: Complexion enhancing tea 贵妃美颜茶

Ingredients: 5 pieces rose buds, 5g jasmine flowers, 2 pieces red dates, 3g wolfberry

Named after legendary beauty Yang Guifei, this tea uses rose buds and jasmine to improve complexion. Red date tonifies qi and wolfberry tonifies liver yin; they also enhance qi flow.

Preparation method: Infuse all ingredients in hot water for 10 minutes.

11.2 Herbs Promoting Blood Flow (活血化瘀药)

Herbs for promoting blood flow and removing stasis are attributed mainly to the liver and heart meridians, and are usually warm, pungent and bitter. They are used to relieve pain and regulate menstruation. Pregnant women and women with heavy menstrual issues, and patients who are on blood thinners or anticoagulants, should use these herbs with caution.

(i) Sichuan lovage root (*chuanxiong* 川芎)
This root is found in Sichuan province in China. It is used extensively in clinical practice.

Therapeutic actions: *Chuanxiong* helps to promote blood and qi flow, and is used to treat pain from cold syndrome causing qi stagnation and blood stasis. It also helps with expelling wind pathogen and is commonly used in prescriptions for rheumatism. *Chuanxiong* is also regarded as an important herb for treating headaches.

Recipe: Fish head soup for headache

Ingredients: One and a half fish head, 5g *chuanxiong*, 5g *tianma*, 5g *baizhi* (白芷), a few pieces of ginger, 3 tablespoons rice wine and oil

Chuanxiong, tianma and *baizhi* are important herbs for relieving headache. As some headaches are due to wind, *baizhi* assists *chuanxiong* in expelling external wind while *tianma* helps to calm internal liver wind. Ginger and wine remove the fishy odour; wine also improves the flow of qi and blood.

Preparation method: Warm the wok, add some oil and stir fry ginger till golden brown. Add the rice wine and fry the fish head for about 2 minutes until slightly brown. Transfer the fish head to a claypot and add the herbs. Add about 1.4 litre of water and a few more pieces of ginger, then cover the claypot. Put the claypot into a bigger pot to double boil for 1.5 to 2 hours.

(ii) Tumeric (*jianghuang* 姜黄)

Tumeric, a member of the ginger family, is the tuber root of the *Curcuma longa* plant. It has recently gained attention in biomedical literature as a source of curcumin, which is used as a remedy for oxidative stress and inflammatory conditions, metabolic syndrome, arthritis, anxiety, hyperlipidemia, exercise-induced inflammation and muscle soreness.[16]

Therapeutic actions: It is one of the few blood promoting herbs that also regulates qi flow. It helps to clear collaterals to relieve pain.

Recipe: Tumeric cauliflower rice 姜黄菜花饭

Ingredients: 4 heads of chopped or grated cauliflower, 2 teaspoons tumeric powder, 1 tablespoon cumin, 1 cup sunflower oil, salt, red pepper flakes, black pepper, cilantro (optional)

Tumeric and cumin both regulate qi flow to relieve pain. Cumin also warms the body and harmonises the stomach, hence it can help with abdominal pain. Cauliflower is easy to digest and good as a replacement of rice. This dish is suitable for people who have bloatedness or pain due to qi stagnation.

---

[16] Hewlings, SJ and Kalman, DS (2017)

Preparation method: Chop the cauliflower into equal sizes (1 inch pieces) and grate them in a food processor with regular blade or grater blade in bursts of a few seconds. Preheat the oven to 220°C. In a small bowl, combine the sunflower oil, cumin, turmeric, red pepper flakes, black pepper and ½ teaspoon of salt. On a baking tray, lay a large rimmed baking sheet. Place the grated cauliflower on the tray and sprinkle spiced oil on it. Toss well then spread the cauliflower evenly to bake for about 1 hour until browned and tender. Sprinkle with cilantro and serve.

(iii) Salvia root (*danshen* 丹参)

The salvia root is also known as red sage or Chinese sage. Clinical studies suggest that *danshen* dilates coronary arteries. It is one of the principal herbs used in *fufang danshendiwan* (复方丹参滴丸) used to treat mild coronary heart disease. Although it primarily promotes blood flow, *danshen* is said to be as powerful a blood tonic as *siwutang* (四物汤).

Therapeutic actions: *Danshen* is cool in nature and in this respect different from other blood flow promoting herbs which are warm. Due to its cool nature, *danshen* has the action of cooling blood to promote healing of abscesses. It also soothes irritability and calms the mind and can be used to treat insomnia arising from blood heat syndrome. Because it promotes better blood circulation, *danshen* is commonly used to treat menstruation problems such as irregularity, cramps, and low menstruation volume. It also removes blood stasis and relieves pain, including chest and abdominal pains.

Recipe: Danshen heart protection wine 丹参护心酒

Ingredients: 30g *danshen*, 15g peach seed, 9g safflower, 500ml Chinese white wine (about 50% alcohol content), one air tight jar

This wine is good for promoting blood flow and preventing ischemic heart disease. Both peach seeds and safflower assist *danshen* in improving blood circulation. Chinese white wine helps to effectively extract the useful constituents of *danshen*.

Preparation method: Put *danshen*, peach seeds and safflower into an air tight jar. Pour in the Chinese white wine and close the lid, and store in cool shaded place. Soak for a month. Take 20ml each time.

(iv) Peach seed (*taoren* 桃仁)

This is the seed of the *Prunus persica (L.) Batsch* or *Prunus davidiana (Carr.) French* species of peach. Peach seed is used with safflower as a pair to promote blood flow. The peach seeds contain amygdalin and should not be taken in excess because of possible cyanide poisoning.

Therapeutic actions: This herb is useful for conditions related to blood stasis, such as menstrual problems, post-partum abdominal pain, lumps, growths, and external injuries. It has similar properties to apricot seeds to moisten the intestine for bowel movement, and to relieve cough and asthma.

Recipe: It is used in *Danshen* heart protection wine mentioned earlier.

(v) Safflower (*honghua* 红花)

Safflower is a spice and a common ingredient for tea. It is a substitute for saffron (*zanghonghua* 藏红花), a more costly ingredient used in French, Indian and Spanish cuisine. The safflower plant is cultivated for vegetable oil and as a source of dye, as well as for medicinal purposes.

Therapeutic actions: Safflower is particularly useful for treating delayed menstruation, menstrual cramp, and post-partum abdominal pain due to blood stasis. It promotes blood flow, removes blood stasis to relieve pain and stimulates menstruation.

Saffron has similar therapeutic actions to safflower but its effect is stronger. In addition, saffron cools the blood and clears toxin, and is especially good for red and inflamed skin.

Recipe: Safflower and argy wormwood leaf footbath 红花艾叶泡脚水
Ingredients: 20g each of safflower and wormwood.

Both safflower and wormwood leaf remove stasis and relieve pain. Wormwood leaf warms the collaterals and disperses cold pathogen to relieve pain.

Preparation method: Rinse and soak the herbs in water for 15 minutes, then boil for 20 minutes. Pour the decoction into a footbath pail. Add more room temperature water to cool it down to about 38°C to 40°C before soaking the feet in the bath for 20 to 30 minutes.

11.3 Hemostatic Herb (止血药)

These are herbs that can stop internal and external bleeding.

Panax notoginseng (*sanqi* 三七)

Sanqi or *tianqi* (田七) is one of the best herbs to stop bleeding. It is an important ingredient in the well known prescription *Yunnan baiyao* (云南白药) for treating injuries due to trauma.

Therapeutic actions Although *sanqi* helps to stop bleeding, it also promotes blood flow to prevent blood stasis. *Sanqi* is also called pseudoginseng because it does not damage *zhengqi* (healthy qi) when promoting blood flow, as most blood flow promoting herbs are inclined to do (which explains why we should avoid prolonged use of other blood flow promoting herbs). *Sanqi* promotes wound healing, reduces bruises and swellings, and relieves pain. It can be taken orally or applied externally for injuries.

Recipe: Sanqi black fungus pork soup 三七木耳炖猪肉

Ingredients: 5g *sanqi* powder, 2 pieces black fungus , 100g sliced pork, spring onion, ginger, salt

This soup is good for people with weak constitutions who have sustained injuries. Pork tonifies blood, while *sanqi* and black fungus promote blood flow for better recovery.

Preparation method: Rinse and soak the black fungus until it is fully expanded. Add sliced pork, black fungus, spring onion, ginger and salt to a pot of water. Double boil for about 2 hours until the pork is soft. Add *sanqi* powder before consuming.

11.4 Astringents (收涩药))

These herbs have an arresting action, they prevent excessive loss of fluids from the body, whether in the form of sweat, urine, stools, discharges, seminal fluids, or blood. Most of them are either sour or astringent in flavour. Generally, these herbs provide symptomatic relief from fluid loss but do not resolve the underlying problem. Hence they should be paired with other herbs that resolve the underlying syndrome. For example, an astringent should be paired with a qi tonic to address excessive sweating due to qi deficiency.

(i) Nutmeg (*roudoukou* 肉豆蔻)

Nutmeg is a spice made from the seed of a tree genus *Myristica*, which is native to Indonesia. It has been a highly treasured spice since the 1st century A.D. Today, it is one of the popular spices in Asian and European cuisines. The processing of nutmeg involves sunning for 6 to 8 weeks until the seed shrinks and rattles upon shaking.

Therapeutic actions: Nutmeg is a warm herb with a distinct strong pungent flavour. It not only warms the spleen and stomach, but also regulates qi. It is very effective in relieving diarrhoea due to spleen yang deficiency or internal cold pathogens through its astringent action on the large intestine. Symptoms of such diarrhoea are chronic watery stools, a feeling of coldness in the abdomen, bloating, and aversion to cold foods or drinks. However, if the diarrhoea is due to heat dampness with symptoms such as strong urge to defecate and foul-smelling yellow stools, burning sensation in the anus, and strong abdominal pain with thirst and irritability, nutmeg should not be used. Although nutmeg is a non-toxic spice, it should not be taken in excess as it may cause allergic reactions such as rashes.

Recipe: Nutmeg pork rib soup 肉豆蔻排骨汤

Ingredients: 2 nutmeg, 8 pieces amomum (*sharen* 砂仁), 20g poria, 300g pork ribs, slices of ginger

This soup warms the spleen and stomach of those who have diarrhoea or bloating due to deficiency cold syndrome. As dampness tends to be formed because of poor functioning of spleen, herbs for resolving dampness are also added in this recipe. This includes amomum, which relieves diarrhoea and bloating by warming the spleen and stomach, and poria, a mild spleen tonic that removes dampness through urination.

Preparation method: Rinse the herbs. Wash the pork ribs and blanch them in hot water. Add 2 litres of water into a pot with pork ribs, ginger and poria. Bring to boil and simmer over low heat for 30 minutes. Add amomum and nutmeg and continue to cook for 15 to 20 minutes and not more because of the volatile nature of the active constituents. Season with salt.

(ii) Lotus seed (*lianzi* 莲子)
In the classic Chinese pharmacopedia by *Sheng Nong,* lotus seed is documented as a good quality herb because of its benefits for attaining longevity. As such, the seeds of the beautiful lotus flower are also known as the fruits of kidney (水中肾果) because the kidney governs ageing. There are two types of lotus seeds. The brown lotus seed is harvested from a ripened seed head. The white lotus seed, with the shell and membranes removed, is harvested when the seed head is still young and green even though the seeds have matured.

Therapeutic actions: Lotus seed is a versatile neutral herb that nourishes several *zang* organs. It strengthens the spleen to relieve diarrhoea, nourishes the heart to calm the mind for better sleep, and tonifies the kidney to slow down ageing. It also prevents abnormal discharges in women and premature ejaculation and involuntary seminal emission in men. The brown lotus seed is better for nourishing the heart, hence it is used in insomnia due to heart qi deficiency. The white lotus seed is stronger for invigorating the spleen, and is used to treat chronic diarrhoea due to spleen qi deficiency.

Recipe: Lotus seed with lily bulb and longan soup 莲子百合龙眼汤

Ingredients: 100g lotus seeds (soak for 30 minutes and remove the embryos), 30g dried longan, 20g dried lily bulb (soak until soft), rock sugar (optional)

This soup suits those who have insomnia due to heart blood and yin deficiency. Longan is a blood tonic that nourishes heart blood and lily bulb is a yin tonic that removes deficiency fire. The embryos of lotus seeds are removed as they are too cooling. The best time to drink this soup is a couple of hours before sleep. It can also be used as a dessert.

Preparation method: Bring 2 litres of water to boil. Add lotus seeds and cook in medium heat for about 30 to 40 minutes or until they have softened. Add lily bulbs and longan meat and cook for another 10 to 15 minutes over low heat. Add rock sugar before serving.

(iii) Gordon seed (*qianshi* 芡实)

The Gordon seed is from the Makhana plant, which is a prickly water lily that originates from Jiangsu province in China. Because of its high nutritional value and health benefits for longevity, it was named the "water ginseng" (水中人参). The poet Su Dong Po reputedly ate 10 to 30 cooked Gordon seeds daily to keep himself in the pink of health.

Therapeutic actions: Gordon seed has similar medicinal properties to lotus seeds. Both are neutral and have tonifying effects on the spleen and kidney to relieve diarrhoea and consolidate essence. They are also used to treat abnormal vaginal discharges in women, as well as involuntary seminal emission in men. However, Gordon seed also removes dampness and can be used to treat chronic diarrhoea resulting from dampness syndrome.

Lotus seed and Gordon seed are considered mild tonics, hence they are safe to consume as food on a regular basis. This is why the formulation *Si Shen Tang* (四神汤), which uses these ingredients, is given to babies and children to strengthen the spleen for a stronger digestive and immune system.

Recipe: Gordon seed pork soup with walnut and Chinese yam 核桃淮山芡实猪展汤

Ingredients: 250g pork shank, 30g walnut, 20g Gordon seed, 20g Chinese yam, 20g wolfberries, 3 candied dates, salt

This nourishing soup can be used for the whole family as it is not too heaty. All the ingredients are neutral in nature with mild tonifying effects on the spleen and kidney. Walnut is a mild kidney tonic that also helps to nourish the brain for better focus and memory.

Preparation method: Rinse the herbs. Blanch the pork shank for 5 minutes and set it aside. Add all ingredients except wolfberries to a pot of water and bring to boil. Cook over low heat for 1 hour. Add wolfberries and continue to simmer for another 10 minutes. Add salt to taste and serve warm.

Chapter 12

Acupuncture and Tuina

During his historic visit to China in 1972, President Nixon witnessed one of the wonders of ancient Chinese science. Surgeries were conducted with acupuncture anaesthesia with patients awake.[17] The drama was not lost on the international television audience, and interest in acupuncture surged in the West. Today acupuncture is practised in almost all advanced Western countries for pain relief as well as a variety of conditions ranging from Bell's Palsy through insomnia to erectile dysfunction. Most treatments are eligible for medical insurance claims.

Numerous scientific studies and clinical trials have shown acupuncture to be effective for many medical complaints, even as debate continues over the validity of some of these studies.[18]

Acupuncture and Tuina (针推) comprise treatment methods based on the TCM meridian system (经络系统). They include acupuncture (*zhen* 针), moxibustion (*jiu* 灸), tuina, cupping (*baguan* 拔罐) and scraping (*guasha* 刮痧).

12.1 History of Acupuncture

Historically, acupuncture began with the use of *bian* stones (砭石), a type of limestone that when pressed or placed warm on certain parts of the body alleviated pain. Later in the Stone Age sharpened stones that pierced the skin (*bianci* 砭刺) were used for treatment. Over several millenia, much advancement was made in techniques

---

[17] See, for example, Wittie (2018)
[18] See, for example, Hong, ed. (2013)

and instruments for acupuncture. Today the use of fine sterile filiform disposable needles is the standard. There are also various devices to enhance needle stimulation through passing small electric currents between needles.

The scope of acupuncture and the meridian system has been gradually expanded over many centuries. 160 acupuncture points identified in *Neijing* were increased to 349 in the *Systemic Classics of Acupuncture and Moxibustion (Zhenjiu Jiayi Jing* 针灸甲乙经).[19] Even in the 20th century, new acupuncture systems like *Dongshi* acupuncture therapy (董氏奇穴疗法) were developed and other new acupoints discovered.

The Chinese term for acupuncture *zhenjiu* (针灸) embodies two related modes of therapy, namely needle acupuncture and moxibustion. Moxibustion is used to warm the body and improve the flow of qi and blood. The combination enhances treatment effect. Infrared lamps can be used in place of heat from moxibustion, although they do not have the medical effect of volatile chemicals in moxibustion smoke that may diffuse into the skin. In this book, acupuncture refers to needle acupuncture.

12.2 The Meridian System

The meridian system forms the diagnostic and treatment framework for acupuncture and tuina. In TCM theory, the meridian system (*jingluo* 经络) is a network of passages through which qi and blood flow. It comprises main trunk routes called the meridians (*jingmai* 经脉) or channels, as well as smaller branches called collaterals (*luomai* 络脉). The meridians run at the level of muscles and organs and are at a deeper level than the collaterals which run just below the skin.

The principal components of the network are the 12 main meridians (十二经脉) and 8 "extraordinary vessels" (*qijing bamai*

---

[19] John C. Longhurst (2010).

Table 12.1   The 12 Main Meridians

Yin Meridians	Zang Organ	Yang Meridians	Fu Organ
Hand *taiyin* 手太阴	Lung 肺	Hand *yangming* 手阳明	Large intestine 大肠
Hand shaoyin 手少阴	Heart 心	Hand *taiyang* 手太阳	Small intestine 小肠
Hand *jueyin* 手厥阴	Pericardium 心包	Hand *shaoyang* 手少阳	Sanjiao 三焦
Foot *taiyin* 足太阴	Spleen 脾	Foot *yangming* 足阳明	Stomach 胃
Foot *shaoyin* 足少阴	Kidney 肾	Foot *taiyang* 足太阳	Bladder 膀胱
Foot *jueyin* 足厥阴	Liver 肝	Foot *shaoyang* 足少阳	Gallbladder 胆

奇经八脉). Each of the 12 main meridians is connected to a particular *zang* or *fu* organ and is named after that organ. The 12 main meridians connect the organs to the exterior of the body. They run through the limbs, head, face and thoracic regions and are distributed symmetrically on each side of the body (Fig. 12.1).

The 8 extraordinary vessels have no direct connection with the organs. The most commonly used extraordinary vessels for therapy are the governor vessel (*dumai* 督脉) and the conception vessel (*renmai* 任脉). Among the 8 extraordinary vessels, only these two have acupuncture points identified along their pathways.

12.3 Acupuncture Points

Each acupuncture point has a specific set of clinical uses. Application of needles or pressure ("acupressure") on these points can have the effect of tonifying, purging, regulating qi and blood flow, warming, or dissipating heat, depending on the needle manipulation techniques used.

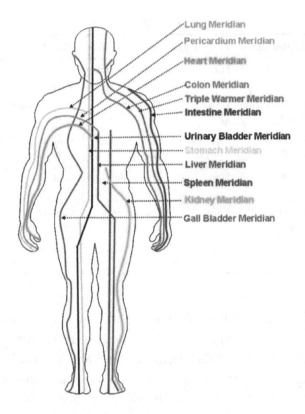

Lung Meridian
Pericardium Meridian
Heart Meridian

Colon Meridian
Triple Warmer Meridian
Intestine Meridian

Urinary Bladder Meridian
Stomach Meridian
Liver Meridian
Spleen Meridian
Kidney Meridian
Gall Bladder Meridian

Fig. 12.1 The twelve main meridians[20]

Acupuncture points may be classified into three categories:

1) **Meridian points** (*jingxue* 经穴) are found along the 12 main meridians, governor vessel and conception vessel. These points have fixed locations and their applications are closely related to their corresponding meridians. For example, most of the points on the conception vessel are used to treat gynecological problems. Points on the kidney meridian have therapeutic effects mainly of strengthening kidney functions.

---

[20] Drake Inner Prizes.com/Energy Medicine (2022)

2) **Extraordinary points** (*qixue* 奇穴) are not located on the 14 meridians. For example, the points *taiyang* (太阳) on our temples are used for ailments such as headache, eye disorders and facial paralysis. In general, the extraordinary points have more specific but narrower applications.

3) ***Ashi* points** (*ashixue* 阿是穴) are tender spots that are not marked by fixed location and do not have any direct relationship with any of the meridians. They do not have specific names and are generally known as *ashi* points as the patient's satisfied cry "Ashi!" suggests a nice response when the needle finds the right spot. They are used mainly in pain treatment as they are located by the physicians based on the areas that are most painful.

Among the acupuncture points used in TCM, some are convenient for applying acupressure on ourselves to promote health. Some common ones are described below.

Hegu (合谷)

Location: At the back of the hand, about halfway between the first and second metacarpals.
Applications: Pain in the facial region (e.g. headache, toothache, sore eyes); external syndromes of coughs and colds. Pregnant women should avoid pressing it.

Neiguan (内关)

Location: Three finger widths up from the inner side of the wrist, between the two tendons.
Applications: Mild angina pain, heart palpitation; digestive disorders such as gastric pain, nausea, vomiting; dizziness, car sickness, migraine; insomnia, depression, stroke, tightness in the chest.

Zusanli (足三里)

Location: Four finger widths down from the center of the depression on the outer side of the knee cap.
Applications: Digestive problems and improving general wellbeing.

Taiyang (太阳)

Location: The head region, one middle finger width away from the outer corner of the eye.
Applications: Headache, eye disorders, facial paralysis.

Baihui (百会)

Location: At the head region. It is the midpoint of the line joining the uppermost tips of the ears.
Applications: Headache, insomnia, stroke, forgetfulness, dizziness.

Shuigou (水沟), also known as *renzhong* (人中)

Location: At the upper one-third point of the philtrum which is the area between the nose and the upper lip.
Applications: Used during emergencies such as fainting, unconsciousness, stroke and epilepsy; also helps nasal congestion.

Fengchi (风池)

Location: It is the depression at the back of the neck below the occipital which is the base of the skull.
Applications: Neck stiffness; internal wind syndromes that may result in stroke, epilepsy, dizziness; external wind syndromes causing colds and nasal congestion. The main therapeutic effect of *fengchi* is to expel wind pathogens.

Guanyuan (关元)

Location: Four finger widths down from the navel.

Applications: Gynecological and andrological disorders; urinary tract disorders; abdominal pain, diarrhea, dysentery, sterility, prolapse of rectum, other intestinal disorders; deficiency due to cold and exhaustion; other conditions due to deficiency of original qi. It has the therapeutic effect of warming the body.

Sanyinjiao (三阴交)

Location: Four finger widths up from the ankle bone protrusion, at the inner part of the leg.

Applications: Digestive disorders; gynecological problems; urinary problems; yin deficiency syndromes. Pregnant women should avoid pressing it.

Taichong (太冲)

Location: At the back of the foot, between the first and second metatarsals.

Applications: Syndromes arise from liver imbalances (liver heat, liver yin deficiency, etc) that result in headache, dizziness, eye redness, and gynecological problems (irregular menses, menstrual cramps, heavy flow).

Shenmen (神门)

Location: Situated on the ulnar side of the wrist and inner side of the tendon.

Applications: Symptoms related to the heart like mental disorders, irritability, shock, anxiety, forgetfulness, insomnia and heart palpitations.

Zhigou (支沟)

Location: Four finger widths up from the outer side of the wrist crease between two bones.
Applications: Constipation; soreness and pain in the shoulder and arm.

Zhongwan (中脘)

Location: At the abdominal area, midpoint between the end of the chest bone and navel.
Applications: Digestive disorders such as abdominal pain and bloatedness, poor appetite, nausea and vomiting.

Tianshu (天枢)

Location: 3 finger widths horizontally from the centre of the navel.
Applications: Gastrointestinal disorders such as abdominal pain and bloatedness, constipation and diarrhoea; gynecological disorders such as irregular menstruation and menstrual cramps.

It has been claimed that pressing the first three points, *zusanli*, *hegu* and *neiguan* regularly has prophylactic health benefits and prevents disease. Acupressure using fingers or a short stick with a rounded end for 15 minutes on each of these points, done two to three times a day, can go some way to strengthen qi, improve flows in the body, strengthen the heart and improve mental agility.

12.4 Acupuncture Points for Common Conditions

Acupuncture points are commonly used in combination like a prescription for illness. Below are some acupoints regularly used by physicians.

i. Post-stroke recovery

Main points: *Neiguan* 内关, *shuigou* 水沟, *sanyinjiao* 三阴交, *jiquan* 极泉, *chize* 尺泽, *weizhong* 委中

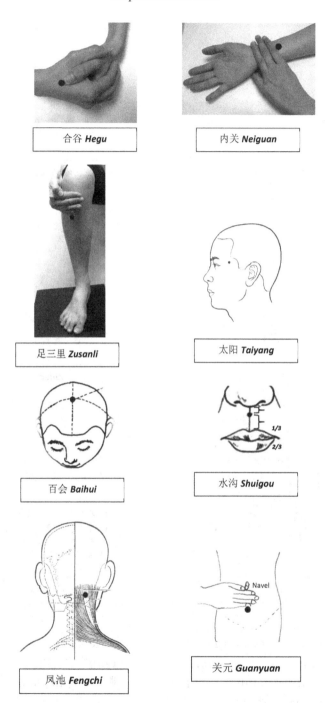

合谷 *Hegu*

内关 *Neiguan*

足三里 *Zusanli*

太阳 *Taiyang*

百会 *Baihui*

水沟 *Shuigou*

凤池 *Fengchi*

关元 *Guanyuan*

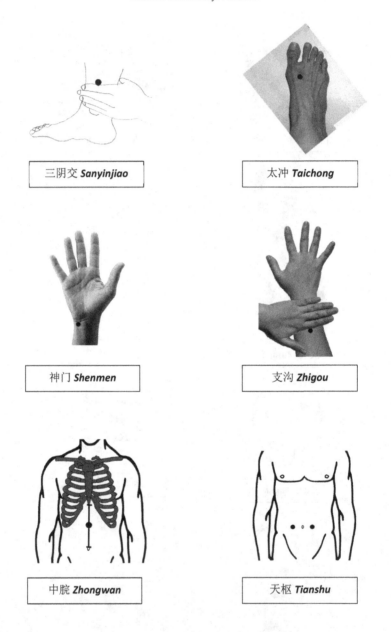

三阴交 *Sanyinjiao*

太冲 *Taichong*

神门 *Shenmen*

支沟 *Zhigou*

中脘 *Zhongwan*

天枢 *Tianshu*

Mouth/face paralysis: *Dicang* 地仓、*jiache* 颊车

Upper limb paralysis: *Jianyu* 肩髃、*shousanli* 手三里、*hegu* 合谷

Lower limb paralysis: *Huantiao* 环跳, *yanglingquan* 阳陵泉, *xuanzhong* 悬钟, *taichong* 太冲

ii. **Insomnia**
   Baihui 百会, *shenmen* 神门, *neiguan* 内关
iii. **Headache**
   Baihui 百会, *fengchi* 风池, *taiyang* 太阳, *hegu* 合谷
iv. **Constipation**
   Zhongwan 中脘, *tianshu* 天枢, *zusanli* 足三里, *zhigou* 支沟

12.5 Moxibustion

Moxibustion uses moxa floss processed from wormwood (mugwort) leaves (艾叶) in tube or fusiform shape, with the smoking end placed above an acupuncture point or over a body area.

The heat from the moxibustion stimulates the acupuncture points and warms the meridians. It also helps to disperse cold pathogen, strengthen the body's yang qi, and resolve blood stasis and stagnation. It also has benefits of disease prevention and health preservation when applied to acupuncture points like *zusanli* and *guanyuan*.

12.6 Tuina

Tuina employs the same therapeutic principles as acupuncture, which are to regulate yin and yang, achieve harmony and balance in the body and stimulate smooth flows of qi and blood by working on the meridians and acupuncture points. Instead of using needles to stimulate the acupuncture points, tuina applies pressure on and/or massages the points along the meridians.

It is important to caution that tuina is different from ordinary massage practised in health spas. Tuina applies TCM theory for therapeutic effects on pain and to treat such conditions as digestive and menstruation disorders, dizziness, anxiety and insomnia.

Child tuina can be performed on children including infants whose health is enhanced by boosting the functions of the organs, especially those of the respiratory and digestive systems, promoting overall growth and development and strengthening bonding between parents and children. It is believed that regular tuina helps to strengthen the child's immune system and wellbeing.

Child tuina requires the application of pressure as for adult tuina, but with less force, on the acupuncture points. A child's acupuncture points are usually not as sharply defined and are in form of areas or zones rather than small points. Furthermore, different areas may be used from those for adults. For example, rubbing the first segment of the child's thumb is equivalent to pressing the *zusanli* on the adult patient. Both have the same effect of strengthening spleen and stomach functions. Lubricants such as talcum powder or baby's oil are necessary in child tuina to reduce friction. The choice of acupuncture points and techniques employed depend on the age, body constitution and underlying syndromes of the patient. This applies equally to adult and child tuina.

12.7 Cupping

Cupping is a form of therapy in which cups are placed on surface of the body. Suction is created either by heating the air in the cups with a flame to create negative pressure, or by pumps that remove air.

The cups are usually placed on acupuncture points or localized area of pain. The typical method of cupping would be to leave the cups for 10 to 15 minutes on the body after suction has been applied. Two other common techniques are gliding the cups along the meridians ("moving cupping") or quickly and repeatedly applying suction with the cups then removing them. This is known as flash cupping.

After cupping, it is normal for the skin to flush red, or have tiny red spots or bruise marks. Some may feel sore, but these side effects would normally go away after a few days.

Cupping has massage-like effect. It helps improve circulation and removes external pathogens. It is usually used for muscle aches, sprains and fever due to cold or flu.

12.8 Scraping (*Guasha*)

Scraping is performed using a tool with smooth edges, like a porcelain spoon or scraping board. The skin is scraped along the meridians at the back of the body in one direction. Scraping is normally done repeatedly until tiny red spots are seen, supposedly indicating that pathogens have been removed from the body. Scraping works like the moving cupping technique. It is often used to reduce fever and improve blood circulation.

Chapter 13

Yangsheng (养生) The Art of Cultivating Life

Since time immemorial man has sought immortality by pursuing the elixir of life. The great emperor *Qin Shi Huang* (秦始皇) subdued all warring states, united all of China under one sovereign for the first time in history, and established the Qin dynasty (221–207 BC). The Qin emperor was held in awe for his military genius and ruthless exercise of power, and could have almost anything he wanted. But one thing eluded him. He ordered his best physicians to scour the earth for the elixir or *xiandan* (仙丹) to cheat death, brutally executing those who failed. The wiliest of his physicians concocted a potion that invigorated him but laced it with enough mercury to kill him slowly. The Qin emperor's only claim to immortality is the enormous underground cavern that houses his hidden tomb, guarded by thousands of terracotta soldiers in the ancient capital of Xian.

The Qin dynasty fell quickly and was succeeded by the glorious Han dynasty, when the great classic *Huangdi Neijing* emerged. It declared that immortality was unattainable. Man had an average life span of 100 years, but most fell short of it because they had not learned to cultivate life, or *yangsheng* (养生).

In modern times, not only have over-stressed city dwellers failed to cultivate life, but their living habits seem almost designed to undermine health and longevity. As Fig. 13.1 illustrates, the progression of man, particularly after the Industrial Revolution in 18th century Europe and the information technology revolution of the late 20th century, has been to violate the natural laws of health.

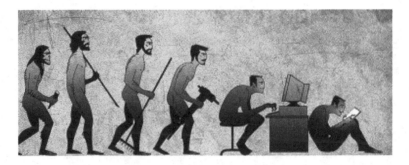

Fig. 13.1   The progression of civilization

Chronic illnesses of modern man are the result of civilization itself that has taken us away from the lifestyle of the hunter gatherer, for which natural evolution had prepared us.[21] Instead, we live sedentary lives, take processed food and synthetic pharmaceuticals, and subject ourselves to continual and unremitting stress.

13.1 The *Neijing* on Cultivating Life

In a celebrated passage on cultivating life, the *Huangdi Neijing* declares:

The ancients knew the *dao* and understood the principles of yin and yang. They practised exercises of body and mind, observed moderation and appropriateness of diet, kept regularity in living habits, and avoided over-exertion. They achieved harmony of body and spirit.[22]

This short passage captures the essence of *yangsheng*. We can summarize it as four principal guidelines:

1. Regularity in living habits (起居有常)
2. Moderate and appropriate diet (饮食有节)

---

[21] Ilardi (2013).
[22] The Chinese text puts it more succinctly: "上古之人，其知道者；法于阴阳，和与术数。饮食有节，起居有常。不妄作劳，故能形与神俱。"

3. Exercises involving breathing techniques (术数)
4. Nourishing mind and spirit (养神)

Regularity in living habits

This comprises rising in the morning and retiring to bed at fixed times according to the seasons, eating regular meals at about the same time, and working hours that follow patterns dictated by the climate and time of the year. Such regularity makes for optimal functioning of the body. It means actively working or exercising when yang qi is abundant in the morning and early afternoon and preparing to rest in the early evening when the yin cycle of the day takes over, reaching a peak at midnight. (See Fig. 4.2 in chapter 4).

The importance of regularity has been noted by Western observers. The greatest of German philosophers Immanuel Kant (1724–1804) was known to be a creature of habit, adhering so religiously to daily schedules that his neighbours would set their clocks according to the time the learned Kant passed their windows on his morning walks. Kant lived to the age of 80, unusual for his generation.

Modern physiologists know that sleeping early allows the body to repair itself efficiently and facilitates the function of the liver. Poor observance of regularity by top executives, missing lunches and dining late as business meetings require, has been speculated to be correlated with their higher incidence of pancreatic cancer among executives with undisciplined schedules. The pancreas is known to be more sensitive to irregular cycles upsetting its sugar regulating functions.[23]

Moderate and appropriate diet

This implies not over-eating (80 percent full is healthier than a full stomach), using moderate quantities of a variety of foods, and

---

[23] Steve Jobs of Apple Inc. arguably may have been a victim of this.

eating the foods appropriate to one's constitution and season of the year. The right diet would include herbs to balance the body, tonics to fortify the *zhengqi* of the body, and herbal supplements that promote the flow of qi, blood and body fluids.

The role of diet in yangsheng

The role of diet in *yangsheng* may therefore be described as follows:

1. Restore normal body functions and overcome deficiencies (扶正补虚). One should therefore use tonics according to deficiency in qi, blood, yin or yang.
2. Purge excess syndromes and eliminate pathogenic factors (泻实祛邪). Excess syndromes include stagnation of qi, blood stasis, and phlegm-dampness.
3. Prevent illness and promote longevity (防病益寿).

When eating, concentrate on eating, chew the food well and try to eat while in a good mood. Taking a gentle stroll after meals helps food go down and digest properly.

People with deficient spleen yang should eat warm cooked foods and avoid cold uncooked food. Those with spleen deficiency and phlegm-dampness should avoid greasy fried foods, and those with asthma and skin allergies should be cautious with seafood. Later in this chapter, we shall explain in more detail how Chinese diets can be customized to the individual body constitution.

Exercises

The exercises of body and mind known as *shushu* (术数) are an ancient art involving subtle movements with meditation, somewhat similar to their modern counterparts found in various form of *qigong* and *taijiquan* exercises.

Qigong 气功

Qigong is the practice of mental and physical skills that integrate body, breath and mind. It involves stretching of the muscles as well as concentration on breathing. Meditation and breathing promote the production and flow of blood and qi and strengthen the internal organs. "*Qi*" in *qigong* refers to the qi of TCM, "*gong*" means skill or technique, hence *qigong* was originally developed as a method of building and moving qi in the body.

There are many forms of *qigong*. These include martial arts *qigong* which aims to strengthen body and master techniques for defense. Daoist *qigong* cultivates mind and body to prolong life. Confucian *qigong* stresses the importance of fostering one's qi to nurture the character and harmonize family and social relations.

Medical *qigong* is the form of *qigong* that aims to prevent and treat disease, preserve health and prolong life. Historically, it evolved as a school of *qigong* by combining the best from various forms of *qigong*. It integrates three aspects of the exercise — movement, breathing and mind.

There are many methods of medical *qigong*. Among the popular ones are the Eight Brocades or *Baduanjin* (八段锦), comprising eight sets of graceful stretching exercises accompanied by breathing synchronized with slow movements. Another school, derived largely from Daoist *qigong* is *Huichungong* (回春功) which literally means recovery of spring (youth). The movements are slow and deliberate, and the practitioner appears to be performing a slow dance.

TCM *qigong* can be used to prevent and assist in curing illnesses including the common cold, insomnia, digestive disorders, cardiovascular diseases, arthritis, and sexual dysfunction. It strengthens qi and promotes its smooth flow. At the same time, the kidney function is improved with tonification of kidney essence and balancing of its yin and yang.

Taijiquan 太极拳

Originally a form of martial art for offence as well as self-defense, many of its moves are lethal when executed fast. It was later adapted as a form of physical and mental training for health benefits, using the breathing and meditation techniques of *qigong*. Thus, it can also be understood as a martial art incorporating *qigong* techniques, executed in slow graceful movements. Combining movement with quiescence, it is sometimes described as "meditation by movement" because of its calming effects on the mind.

Taijiquan has the additional benefit over most *qigong* exercises: it promotes physical balance, as many movements are executed with only one foot on the floor. Hence it is encouraged as a gentle form of exercise that can help to prevent falls among the elderly. Even the

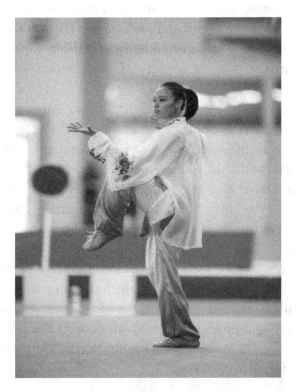

Fig. 13.2   *Taijiquan* promotes balance

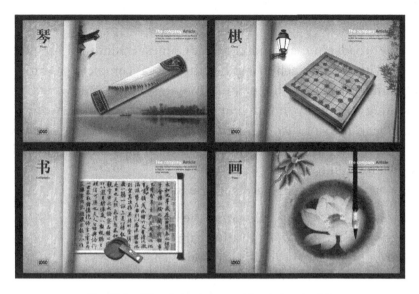

Fig. 13.3 *Qin, qi, shu, hua* nourish mind and spirit

venerable Harvard Medical School promotes it for developing *Taiji* practitioners to be "strong as an oak, flexible as a willow, and mentally clear as still water."[24]

Nourishing mind and spirit

The *Neijing*'s most important instruction is arguably that of maintaining healthy mind and spirit, working smoothly in harmony with the body. Over several millennia, the Chinese have developed many ways of promoting mind and spirit. The Chinese leisure pursuits of the cultured man, comprising calligraphy, painting, playing the musical instrument *qin*, and chess are means of attaining such alertness within serenity.

---

[24] Harvard Medical School (2018) "An Introduction to Tai Chi," Harvard Health Publishing, p3.

13.2 *Yangsheng* Cultivates Life, Not Just Health

On the broader human landscape, the Chinese tradition of *yangsheng* is not just about achieving health, but a complete culture of attaining spiritual fulfilment and happiness deeply intertwined with attaining a healthy mind and body. In the Chinese word for *yangsheng*, the word *yang* 养 means cultivate, and *sheng* 生 means life. *Yangsheng* is more than the cultivation of health: it is the cultivation of life itself.

Yangsheng has many facets. These include:

yangshen	养身	cultivating the body
yangxin	养心	cultivating calm and tranquillity
yangxing	养性	cultivating one's character
yangshen	养神	cultivating the spirit

In some ways, the pecking order in the above list reflects the difficulty of each level of cultivation. Cultivating the body is the easiest, whilst attaining a cultivated spirit is the hardest and most elusive.

Cultivating the body or *yangshen* 养身 involves appropriate nutrition, regularity in living habits, getting enough exercise, and avoiding harmful environmental influences like harsh weather.

To *yangxin* 养心 is cultivate calm and tranquillity. This requires both nurturing the physical health of our heart as an organ involved in calming the mind and enabling sound sleep, but also savouring the freshness of a nature walk, or relaxing by the cool waters of a mountain stream. Worldwide interest in mindfulness and meditation is a healthy trend and reflects the need for people living in stressful environments to *yangxin*. Meditation was shown at Harvard in the 1960s to have salutary effects on our nervous systems, in particular the parasympathetic nervous system with neurotransmitters like serotonin and dopamine to help the body cope with stress and calm the nerves. This in turn has salutary effects on a broad range of conditions like hypertension, gastric disorders and cardiovascular disease.[25]

Cultivating character or *yangxing* 养性 is an important value in Chinese culture, emphasised particularly by Confucian ethics that stresses education and training from a young age to appreciate and practise the virtue of kindness and consideration for others.

The virtues of kindness and benevolence toward others may not appear to be much related to health of the body, but modern psychologists are finding out what the ancients knew all along, that a kind and compassionate heart is good for health of mind and body. For example, Thupten Jinpa argues that a compassionate heart over time can alter the physiology of our brains to make it more resilient and able to deal with anxiety and depression.[26]

Finally, *yangshen* 养神 or cultivation of the spirit is the hardest but most rewarding of all. Each person may have a different path to it. Some achieve it through religion and prayer, others through art and music, and yet others through creative activities that give sustenance to their deeper selves. Daoist philosophers were among the masters of cultivating the spirit. The Chinese art of calligraphy and brush painting, the playing of musical instruments like the *qin*, and the appreciation of arts, are activities that lift the human spirit to a level even higher than that of "self-actualisation" that Maslow placed at the apex of a pyramid of human needs.

13.3 Illness, Ageing and Longevity

Avoiding Illness

A famous passage from the *Neijing* concerns the avoidance of illness:

---

[25] Herbert Benson and his colleagues at Harvard Medical School did extensive studies in the 1960s that established the scientific basis for the medical benefits of meditation. See Benson H and Klipper M Z (1975).

[26] Jinpa (2015).

If you avoid climatic stresses, live a placid life with plain needs, maintain defensive forces in the body, and keep yourself in good spirits, how then could you possibly fall ill?[27]

This passage places the responsibility of disease prevention squarely on each person's own lifestyle and attitude to life. In simple terms: lead a placid life and keep good spirits.

A placid life with plain needs is conducive to avoiding the effects of excessive contemplation and anxiety on the spleen and liver. Digestive problems like acid reflux, bloated stomachs, loss of appetite, stomach ulcers and the irritable bowel syndrome are common in high achievement-oriented societies. Modern treatment with antacids, proton pump inhibitors and drugs to reduce inflammation and excessive gastric secretions only control the symptoms but do not address the underlying causes. To alleviate these conditions, TCM would attack these problems at the level of their syndromes like impeded flows of liver qi and deficiency of spleen qi that in turn may have their origins in stress.

The ageing process

Biomedicine explains that human beings have built-in mechanisms for physiological processes to decline as we get older. Much of it has to do with the ability of cells in the body to regenerate. The telomere at the end of a chromosome, which ensures cell replication, shortens as we age.[28] Replication of telomeres is directed by the enzyme telomerase. Hence ageing to some extent can be mitigated by supplementing the body's telomerase. Drugs like resveratrol extracted from red wine as well as Chinese herbs like astragalus (*huangqi*) can provide this supplementation.

The body's immune system undergoes age-dependent decline. Lymphocytes from older adults have less ability to multiply. The neurological system weakens as neurons do not replicate and older

---

[27]"虚邪贼风, 避之有时, 恬淡虚无, 真气从之, 精神内守, 病安从来。"
[28]Oxford (2007).

ones die.[29] These biological changes are accompanied by physiological declines. Cardiac output is reduced, the elasticity of lung decreases, there is a greater tendency to develop metabolic syndrome. Fluid and electrolyte homeostasis are affected, and vision and hearing suffer neurological decline. Inflammation, which involves oxidative stress, further disrupts the immune system and encourages the development of chronic illnesses like diabetes, arthritis and cardiovascular diseases. Quantum leaps in achieving longevity must come from methods that directly intervene in the ageing process. Recent promising developments include those proposed in David Sinclair's popular book *Lifespan*.[30]

From the TCM point of view, ageing results in the weakening of the *zang* organs. The spleen has more difficulty in transforming food and the body becomes more vulnerable to attack by external pathogens. A weak qi constitution can succumb to infection that develops into excess heat syndrome. It becomes harder to treat with heat-clearing herbs as many of these herbs may also weaken qi. Ageing invariably increases blood stasis and phlegm retention, which can affect moods and stir up wind. There is a general decline in healthy qi (*zhengqi*) and essence (*jing*) in the kidneys.

At middle age, the average person may look good on the outside but internal organs, qi and blood would be declining. As advanced age sets in, the body develops deficiency in qi and blood. Essence becomes depleted. Blood stasis and turbid phlegm worsen. After retirement, decline in social status can affect self-esteem of the elderly and consequently weaken the organs further.

Coping with ageing

These inevitable consequences of ageing are discouraging but following *yangsheng* principles can ameliorate them and enable us to remain active up to near the end of life.

---

[29] Abrass (1990).
[30] Sinclair (2019).

For the middle-aged, it is important to start cultivating mind and spirit for tranquility. To avoid the onset of serious chronic illnesses, it is necessary to work moderately whilst creating more space for recreation and exercises like walking, biking, *taijiquan* and *qigong*.

Neijing's advice to keep regularity in living habits and avoiding overstrain takes on added urgency. Sexual excesses become less affordable as one's level of qi, essence, and yin or yang become partly depleted. The judicious use of tonics at this stage of life is needed.

As we move into the elderly phase, it is important to attain a certain level of internal equanimity and come to terms with the inevitability of death. We seek peace of mind and adopt a positive outlook through activities that stimulate a passion for living. The company of good friends, appreciation of nature, and stimulating the mind through life-long learning all contribute to longevity.

Diet and exercises must adapt to the reality of a weakened spleen and stomach. It would be prudent to limit or avoid the consumption of cold or uncooked food. Eat warm cooked food that is easy to digest and choose medicated diet over medicine. Gentle exercises should aim to boost qi rather than muscular strength or cardiovascular performance. Tonics should be taken regularly, but only in smaller quantities and spread over longer periods.

13.4 The Blue Zones and *Yangsheng*

In special regions of the world known as the "Blue Zones", there is an unusually high proportion of centenarians living active healthy lives right up to the final months of their lives. A consistent pattern can be seen. They are at peace with plain and simple lives in socially supportive communities where family and friends gather daily to share their joys and worries. There is a warm sense of belonging to a close-knit group.[31]

---

[31] Buettner (2008). We have included Bama, in guanxi Province, China, that was not covered in Buettner's study.

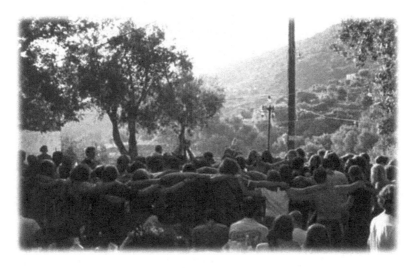

Fig. 13.4　Ikarians dance and sing every day after work

One of the blue zones, the Greek island of Ikaria, is even known as the island where "people forget to die." Each evening, the island's carefree inhabitants meet in the public square to dance and sing, enjoy hearty laughter and conversation, and strengthen communal bonds.

There is no magic common diet in the blue zones. Okinawans feast on pork, Seven Day Adventists in Loma Linda are vegetarians, and Ikarians live on a Mediterranean diet. Interestingly, but perhaps not surprisingly, the lifestyles of inhabitants of the blue zones follow quite closely the prescriptions of the *Neijing* for *yangsheng* (Table 13.2)

13.5　On Diets and Body Constitutions

TCM advocates that diet should be customised to the individual. Our nutritional needs vary according to our constitutions. TCM classifies people as belonging to one of nine kinds of constitution (Table 13.3).

Table 13.2   Blue Zone Lifestyles are in Accord with *Yangsheng*

Blue zone lifestyles compared with *Yangsheng*

Sardinia, Okinawa, Loma Linda (California), Costa Rica, Ikaria, Greece, Bama (Guangxi)
World's highest rate of centenarians; 1 in 3 live past 90 in good health

BLUE ZONES	TCM YANGSHENG
Regular schedules facilitate communal activities	Regularity in living habits; interactions through board games, music
Physically active, not necessarily with vigorous cardiovascular exercises.	Qigong exercises for nurturing *qi*, flow and spirit. Nature walks
Low stress levels	Plain needs; no driving ambitions
No common diet. Varies from vegetarian to mostly meat	Diet fits individual constitution and climatic environment
Mentally and spiritually active. Singing, dancing, close communal interactions delay dementia and infirmity	Calligraphy, painting, chess, music - - keeps the mind and spirit youthful even in old age

Table 13.3   The Nine Kinds of Constitution

TCM Classification of Constitutions

Constitution		Characteristics
Balanced and Harmonius	平和体质	Healthy with no symptom
Qi deficiency	气虚体质	Soft voice, fatigue, spontaneous sweating
Blood deficiency	血虚体质	Pale complexion without lustre, pale lips, dizzy
Yang deficiency	阳虚体质	Aversion to cold, pale complexion
Yin deficiency	阴虚体质	Skinny, facial flush, dry mouth, vexation
Phlegm-Dampness	痰湿体质	Fat, sluggish, soft stools
Damp-Heat	湿热体质	Feverish, aversion to heat, foul soft stools
Qi stagnation	气郁体质	Easily agitated or depressed, chest tightness
Blood stasis	血瘀体质	Dark and dull complexion, dark lips

The first category, the balanced and peaceful constitution, represents the ideal healthy constitution. All the remaining eight constitutions have one or more syndromes, and each person having one of these constitutions is deemed to be not totally well. If the person has no clear clinical symptoms of disease, he is considered to be only sub-clinically ill or *yajiankang*, as described in Chapter 3 of the book. People in these categories need to consume foods that help to correct their imbalances or improve flow within their bodies. Each other type of body constitution has its own set of defining symptoms.

Individuals who have a qi deficiency constitution are often characterized by weakness in the lung and spleen, and present symptoms such as a soft voice, fatigue, spontaneous sweating and poor appetite.

Blood deficiency constitution comes with a pale complexion without lustre, pale lips, dizziness, heart palpitation or early thinning/dropping of hair.

The manifestations of yang deficiency constitution are aversion to cold, frequent night urination (nocturia) and a pale complexion. People with yin deficiency have facial flush, dry mouth and throat, and are easily vexed; more often than not, they are thin.

Phlegm dampness and damp heat body constitutions tend to show symptoms associated with the spleen and stomach because these organs are the main sources for the production of phlegm and dampness. Typical symptoms for a phlegm dampness constitution are plumpness, sluggishness, soft stools and sputum in the morning. For the damp heat constitution, there is aversion to heat, foul and sticky soft stools, a bloated stomach, and oily skin or scalp.

Qi stagnation and blood stasis constitutions commonly experience tightness or body pain as flows are impeded. With the qi stagnation, a person is easily agitated or depressed and may experience chest tightness, whereas for blood stasis constitutions, the complexion is dark and dull, and lips are dark coloured.

Diet and constitution

An individual's constitution is related to their natural long-term underlying syndrome(s). A person with qi weakness should have a

Table 13.4   Tonic Foods for Deficiency Syndromes

Qi tonic foods	Rice, soybean, Chinese yam (*huaishan*), peanuts, *biandou* (扁豆 hyacinth bean), millet, potato, carrot, date, quail and chicken eggs, chicken, beef
Blood tonic foods	pork liver, lamb, beef, sea cucumber, red dates, blackstrap molasses, black fungus, spinach, carrot, *danggui*, dried longan
Yang tonic foods	mutton, shrimp, walnut, Chinese chives, sword bean
Yin tonic foods	white fungus, mulberry fruit, bird's nest, pear, wolfberry seeds, turtle, black sesame seeds, duck, chicken and duck eggs, milk products

Table 13.5   Warm and Cool Foods

Hot/warm foods	mutton, chicken, pork liver, eel, prawn, glutinous rice, longan, lychee, onion, garlic, chives, ginger, chilli, pepper, brown sugar, spring onion, coriander leaf
Cold/cool foods	duck, beef, pork, snakehead fish (*yusheng*), seaweed, kelp, mung bean, bitter gourd, lettuce, bamboo shoots, banana, persimmon, pear, bean curd, milk, wheat, mulberry fruit, apple, water chestnut, red bean, radish, lotus root, Chinese cabbage, tomato,
Neutral foods	chicken egg, carp, yellow croaker, cuttle fish, pigeon, jelly-fish skin, white fungus, pea, lotus seed, Chinese yam, spinach, carrot, white sugar, peanut, soybean, rice, honey, sweet potato, mandarin orange, black fungus, spinach

diet that has qi tonics like soybean and Chinese yam incorporated in it, and one with yin weakness would benefit from a diet with foods that nourish yin, like lily bulb, wolfberry and white fungus (Table 13.4)

A person whose constitution inclines him toward having heat should reduce warm foods and increase consumption of cooler foods (Table 13.5)

Those with excess syndromes or pathogenic factors can be guided by Table 13.6[32,33]

---

[32] Source: Liu and Ma (2007).
[33] 谢梦洲 （主编）(2016).

Table 13.6　Foods for Excess Syndromes or the Presence of Pathogenic Factors

Foods for expelling exogenous pathogens	ginger, shallot, fermented soybean
Foods for clearing internal heat	bitter gourd, bitter vegetables, watermelon, *jue-cai* (蕨菜), water chestnut
Foods for clearing heat dampness	Chinese barley, purslane
Foods for warming the interior	dried ginger, Chinese cinnamon, pepper, mutton, fenne seeds
Foods for regulating qi	sword bean, rose
Foods for promoting blood flow and removing stasis	hawthorn, wine, vinegar
Foods for removing phlegm	marine alga (海藻) kelp, laver (紫菜), sea tangle (海带), turnip, apricot seed
Foods for relieving cough	apricot seed, pear, ginkgo, loquat, lily
Foods for alleviating anxiety	lotus seeds, wheat, longan meat, lily bulb
Foods for promoting bowel movement	apricot seed, prune, black sesame, banana, spinach, bamboo shoot
Food for relieving diarrhea	dark plum, lotus seed

Combining Western and Chinese wisdom in diet

Western nutritionists rightly point out that one should avoid high glycemic index carbohydrates and trans fats, moderate the amount of saturated fats, and eat more vegetables especially those rich in fibre. The Mediterranean diet based on generous amounts of vegetables and nuts combined with moderate amounts of seafood and meat comes close to present Western thinking on the ideal diet, particularly for cardiovascular health.

It is possible to combine this Western wisdom with that of Chinese *yangsheng* by choosing the foods in the Mediterranean diet that suit one's body constitution. For example, a person with qi and blood deficiency weakness can still consume Mediterranean food choices that also have qi and blood tonic effects like Chinese

Table 13.7   Incorporating *Yangsheng* Principles in a Mediterranean Diet

Combining Mediterranean and Chinese diets:

A Mediterranean diet is followed, but the choices of food differ according to person's (TCM) constitution

Example 1: A person with weak *qi* and blood (pale, afraid of cold, thready pulse)	Example 2: A person with yin deficiency (thirsty, warm hands and feet, dry eyes, hot flashes, night sweats)
Carbos: Chinese yam, millet, peanuts	**Carbos**: buckwheat, beehoon, rice porridge
Veges and fruits: peanuts, raisins, spinach, red dates, longan, walnut, almonds	**Veges and fruits**: white fungus, black sesame, water cress, bitter gourd, black beans
Meats: chicken, pork liver, sea cucumber	**Meats**: duck, turtle, bird's nest
Alcohol: rice wine, yellow wine, red wine	**Alcohol**: beer, light white wine, apple cider
Teas: oolong, pu'er	**Teas**: green tea, jasmine, chrysanthemum
Herbs: astragalus (*huangqi*), *danggui*, Chinese yam, **Chinese ginseng**	**Herbs**: wolfberry, lily bulb, *yuzhu*, *maidong*, **American ginseng**

yam, red dates and pork liver, and drink warm (oolong) tea and red wine. However, a person with yin deficiency would choose cooler vegetables and meats and drink green tea and white wine (Table 13.7).

Chapter 14

Medicated Foods and Teas for *Yangsheng*

The renowned Tang dynasty physician Sun Simiao opined that the foundation of body health lay in food: "He who does not understand food is ill-suited to living."[34] Since ancient times, diet has been accorded prime importance in life cultivation. In particular, a diet that is not tailored to the individual person's constitution would be potentially harmful to health.

14.1 Characteristics of Medicated Food

Medicated food, also known as *yaoshan* (药膳), has herbs added to enhance its nutritional value, cooked in such a way as to be delicious and appetising. It accords with the principle that herbs and food come from the same source (*yaoshi tongyuan* 药食同源). The *Neijing* puts it this way: "If it is eaten on an empty stomach when one is well, it is considered as food. If it is eaten when one is unwell, it is regarded as a medicine." (空腹食之为食物，患者食之为药物.)

Medicated diet must take into account the particular syndromes that might be present at the time it is taken. Less seasoning is usually used. Most medicated diets are suitable for long-term consumption. Their therapeutic actions are milder than those of medicinal decoctions as the dosage of herbs used is much lower. To absorb as much nutrients as possible from the food, medicated dishes are

---

[34] (孙思邈) (581–682 A.D).

usually prepared using cooking methods such as boiling, simmering, braising and steaming. These ways of cooking require the dish to be cooked over low heat for longer periods of time to ensure that the nutritious ingredients of the foods are extracted. This explains why most medicated dishes come in the form of soups and porridges with all the goodness of the food ingredients locked in.

The medicated diet is both an art and a science. Many famous recipes have been improved over time by culinary specialists. The science of medicated diets draws on conventional Chinese medical principles. However, compared to medical herbs, the medicinal properties of different foods have not been as well researched and documented. Hence, one should use the information in this chapter only as a guide, even though such information has served the Chinese people well over many generations.

Food Ingredients

As with herbs, foods have their own natures and flavours and generally one should try to have a balance of hot and cold foods. Food that is too hot damages *yin* fluids, and food that is too cold can harm yang qi, especially that of spleen and kidney.

For the medicated food to be nutritious, it is important to adhere to TCM principles. As with prescriptions, each of the ingredients has a role to play whether it is a monarch, minister, adjuvant or guiding role, and the choice of ingredients in the dish is dependent on the syndrome(s) that the dish is addressing. Besides taking into account the therapeutic effects of the ingredients, the taste of the combination of herbs and food ingredients is an important factor for the selection of ingredients.

The therapeutic actions of foods can be classified into tonics to address deficiency syndromes and foods for removing pathogens to treat excess syndromes.

Some examples of foods with warm/cool properties, tonic benefits, and the ability to remove pathogens to treat excess syndromes were provided in Tables 13.4 to 13.6 in the last chapter.

We provide some examples of three kinds of medicated food: porridges, soups and teas. Medicated food of course is available also in other forms such fried, steamed or broiled dishes.

14.2 Porridges

Porridge therapy (*zhouliao* 粥疗) is used in *yangsheng* as well as for treatment of illnesses. Porridge has the special characteristic that rice after long boiling in watery form is easily digestible, hence is suitable for both healthy adults as well as children, the elderly and the sick. Rice, the main ingredient of porridge, is a mild qi tonic, and when porridge is served warm, it harmonizes the stomach, tonifies the spleen, and clears the lung.

There are two main kinds of rice used. These are *jingmi* (粳米) or round-grained rice and *nuomi* (糯米) or polished glutinous rice. *Jingmi* is excellent for nourishment and development, while *nuomi* is ideal for warming and tonifying the stomach. In the old days, most porridges used *jingmi*, although long-grained rice was sometimes used as a substitute and has similar therapeutic actions.

Below are three porridge recipes which incorporate the use of Chinese herbs for different therapeutic effects.

Nourishing yin: Lily and wolfberry porridge (百合枸杞粥)

Ingredients: 30g fresh lily bulb, 30g wolfberry seeds, 100g *jingmi*, olive oil, and spring onions

This porridge nourishes yin of the kidney, liver and lung and also clears eyesight, improves production of fluids, and alleviates (dry) coughs.

Preparation method: Boil rice for 1 hour. Fry the lily bulb in olive oil in a deep pan. Add boiled porridge and wolfberry seeds to the pan, boil and simmer for 30 minutes. Add salt, pepper and spring onion to taste.

Strengthening spleen and stomach: Chinese yam and *dangshen* porridge (山药党参粥)

Ingredients: 30g fresh Chinese yam cut into small chunks (less if dry yam is used), 10g *dangshen* 党参 (sliced), 60g *jingmi* rice, a few slices of lean pork and egg white (optional)

This porridge helps to nourish the spleen and stomach and strengthen their functions, thereby alleviating poor digestion and dyspepsia. It can be an ideal daily breakfast for those with weak spleen and stomach.

Preparation method: Boil rice 1 hour. Add Chinese yam and *dangshen* and continue cooking for 1 hour. Add sliced pork for a quick boil, then add the egg white. Add salt and pepper to taste.

Tonifying kidney yang: Chestnut porridge (栗子粥)

Ingredients: 10–15g chestnut (cut into small chunks), 100g *jingmi* rice, 10–20g wolfberry seeds (optional).

This porridge strengthens the kidney function by tonifying yang. Chestnut has the nickname "fruit of kidney" (肾之果), hence because is suitable for those who have weak kidney functions with aversion to cold and lower backaches. However, because of its warm nature, it should be avoided by people with internal heat. The addition of wolfberry seeds not only gives the porridge a sweet taste, but also provides a tonifying effect on liver and kidney yin, thereby enhancing the action of strengthening kidney functions.

Preparation method: Boil rice for 30 minutes. Add chestnut and continue cooking for 30 minutes to 1 hour until the chestnut is soft. Add wolfberry seeds during the last 10 to 15 minutes. Serve warm.

14.3 Soup Recipes

Soups are generally regarded as nutritious food because nutrients are infused in it after boiling and simmering for hours. As such, it is a good practice to drink soup slowly and before meals so as to allow efficient absorption of nutrients, especially for the case of medicated diets with their therapeutic effects. We briefly describe below some simple recipes for different body constitutions, which you can try out at home. These recipes are just a guide to the types of ingredients to use for the various types of body constitutions or syndromes. You may find it interesting to modify the recipes to make them more appealing to your taste!

Clearing heat and dampness: Job's tears and green bean soup (苡仁绿豆汤)

Ingredients: 100g Job's tears (*yiyiren* 薏苡仁), 50g green beans (绿豆), 5–10g dried tangerine peel (*chenpi* 陈皮)

This soup is suitable for those who have a heat dampness body constitution (湿热体质). It helps to expel toxins, clear summer heat and resolve dampness. The dosage of Job's tears (monarch herb) is the highest as its action of clearing heat dampness is the strongest. Dried tangerine peel is used sparingly because of its bitter taste; it acts as an adjuvant by promoting the flow of qi which is often impeded by dampness. Dried tangerine peel also helps to protect the spleen and stomach from the cool nature of Job's tears and green beans which clear heat but can also hurt the spleen, which is sensitive to cold. A person who has a weak spleen and stomach should avoid drinking this soup. For those who prefer the dish to be more filling, we can add more Job's tears or green beans to make it more like porridge.

Preparation method: Soak Job's tears and green beans in water for at least an hour. Add dried tangerine peel, put them in a pot and add water (about 1500ml). Cook until Job's tears and green beans turn soft. If preferred, you may add some rock sugar for a sweeter taste. Serve warm.

Resolving dampness and phlegm: Gordon seed, lotus seed and Job's tears soup (芡实莲子苡仁汤)

Ingredients: 300g pork ribs (chopped into small chunks), 20g lotus seeds 莲子, 30g gordon fruit (*qianshi* 芡实), 30g Job's tears, 5g dried tangerine peel 陈皮, 1 ginger

This soup helps to resolve dampness and phlegm, and is therefore suitable for those who have a phlegm dampness body constitution (痰湿体质). Gordon seed has the action of removing dampness and lotus seeds help to tonify the spleen so that it will prevent the production of phlegm and dampness. As compared to Job's tears and green bean soup, this soup is not as cooling. It also has a harmonizing effect on the spleen and stomach functions because of the presence of lotus seeds, gordon seed and dried tangerine peel. This soup suits most people because it is milder and the coolness of Job's tears is mitigated by the warm nature of the ginger and dried tangerine peel. Pork ribs are added to enhance the taste of the soup. As gordon seed has an arresting (astringent) action, those inclined to constipation should avoid this dish.

Preparation method: Soak lotus seeds, gordon fruit, Job's tears and dried tangerine peel in water. After soaking, put the pork and herbs in a claypot. Add water and ginger. Bring to boil. Continue to simmer for 2 hours. Add salt to taste. Serve warm.

Promoting blood flow: Chinese angelica, *tianqi* and black chicken soup (当归田七乌鸡汤)

Ingredients: 1 black chicken, 15g Chinese angelica root (*danggui* 当归), 5g *tianqi* 田七, 1 piece ginger (optional)

This soup helps to promote blood flow, remove stasis and nourish blood. It is suitable for those who have a blood stasis body constitution (瘀血体质). Black chicken is a tonic food for qi and blood. *Tianqi* promotes blood flow and removes stasis without damaging the qi in the body. This soup is warm and not suitable for those who have a heat syndrome. Ginger can be removed if this soup tastes too hot. Individuals who have yin deficiency and weak stomachs should avoid taking this soup.

Preparation method: Soak *tianqi* and Chinese angelica root. Put black chicken and the rest of the ingredients into a pot. Add salt and just enough water to cover the black chicken. Double boil on high heat for 3 hours.

Black chicken soup for nourishing blood (养血乌鸡汤)

Ingredients: Black chicken 乌鸡, 10g Chinese angelica root (*danggui* 当归), 20g astragalus (*huangqi* 黄芪), 6g *chuanxiong* 川芎, 10g *shengdihuang* 生地黄, 10g red dates (*dazao* 大枣)

This soup is suitable for individuals who have a blood deficiency constitution (血虚体质). It nourishes blood and also mildly promotes blood flow with the addition of *chuanxiong*. Although *astragalus* is a qi tonic, it is added to assist in the production of blood, since qi is required to produce blood. *Shengdihuang* with its cool nature, is added to mitigate the warming nature of the soup ingredients and has a mild action in nourishing yin. This soup is not as warm as *Bazhen Tang* (八珍汤), and can also be used for women who have just finished menstruation to help replenish blood. Individuals who have heat syndrome should avoid this soup.

Preparation method: Soak all the herbs in 2000ml of water. Blanch the black chicken and put into the pot of water. Bring it to boil and continue to cook it over low heat for another 45–60 minutes. Add salt to taste. Serve warm

Soup for nourishing *yin* (沙参玉竹鸭肉汤)

Ingredients: 600g duck (cut into big pieces), 50g *beishashen* 北沙参, 50g *yuzhu* 玉竹, 2 pieces ginger

This soup nourishes yin, especially lung and stomach yin, and is good for those who have a yin deficiency body constitution (阴虚体质). Duck nourishes yin, and *beishashen* and *yuzhu* are both *yin* tonics, promoting the production of fluids. This soup is good for prevention of dry throat and cough, especially during autumn in temperate countries, as it helps to nourish and moisten the lung. With the addition of ginger, which helps to warm the spleen and stomach, this soup is not as cooling and it can be consumed by most people.

Preparation method: Soak both *beishashen* and *yuzhu* in 2000ml of water for 30 minutes. Add the duck and bring it to a boil. Lower the heat, skim fat from the surface of the soup and continue to simmer for about 30 minutes. Serve warm.

Black bean soup for tonifying kidney (黑豆干貝山药湯)

Ingredients: 10g *duzhong* 杜仲, 50g black beans (soak for 1 hr), 200–250g fresh Chinese yam (*shanyao* 山药) (cut into cubes), 50g red dates (*dazao* 大枣), 30–50g scallop, 30ml rice wine

The main therapeutic action of this soup is to tonify kidney yang, hence it is suitable for yang deficiency body constitution (阳虚体质). Both *duzhong* and black beans tonify yang and strengthen the kidney. Chinese yam nourishes the spleen and kidney. This soup takes care two of the more important *zang* organs in Chinese medicine: the prenatal basis of life (the kidney) and the post-natal basis of life (the spleen). Strengthening the kidney helps prevent premature greying of hair and hair loss.

Preparation method: Add *duzhong*, black beans and scallop into 1500ml of water. Boil over low heat for 1 hour. Add red dates and Chinese yam. Cook for another 5 minutes. Add rice wine and salt to taste. Serve warm.

Strengthening qi: Chicken soup for qi (参芪鸡汤)

Ingredients: 200g Chicken, 15g *dangshen* 党参, 10g astragalus (*huangqi* 黄芪), 100–150g fresh Chinese yam (*shanyao* 山药) (cut into cubes).

Chicken improves qi, hence this soup is for qi deficiency body constitution (气虚体质). In addition, the soup contains qi tonics such as *dangshen, astragalus* and Chinese yam to enhance the replenishing of qi, especially that of the spleen and the lung. This is important since spleen is the source of qi production and lung governs qi. This soup is good for those who tend to feel weak. It is also a dish which can be cooked for the whole family once in a while to replenish qi.

Preparation method: Soak the herbs in 1500ml of water for 30 minutes. Add the blanched chicken and bring it to boil. Add the fresh Chinese yam and continue to simmer over low heat for 30 to 50 minutes. Add salt to taste. Serve warm.

14.4 Herbal Teas

As for medicated food, herbal teas are also customised to the body's condition. The herbs used are mostly of plant origin as they generally taste better and are easier for the extraction of the desired ingredients. Depending on the plant parts, certain herbal teas can easily be made by infusing them in hot water whereas others may need boiling. Herbs that are flowers, leaves or fleshy fruits can be used for infusions, while roots, bark, stems and seeds usually require some boiling.

Unless it is required by your body condition, it is not advisable to drink the same herbal tea daily. It should be taken in moderation and stopped when one feels better, especially for cooling herbal teas as they may harm the spleen and stomach with prolonged use. An exception can be made for teas that are neutral in nature and have tonifying effects. These can be taken more regularly, such as two to three times a week.

Below are a few tantalizing herbal teas recipes for your enjoyment. The quantity of herbs used is for 1 teapot serving.

Clear Vision Tea (清热明目茶)

Ingredients: 8g chrysanthemum flower, 3–6g mulberry leaves, 3–6g wolfberry seeds

As it clears liver fire to improve vision, this tea is ideal for those who stay up late at night and suffer from dry and reddened eyes due to liver fire. Chrysanthemum flowers and mulberry leaves help to clear liver fire while wolfberry seeds nourish liver yin. Some red dates can be added to give the tea a natural sweet taste. As this tea is cooling, it is advisable not to take it for too long.

Preparation method: Steep the herbs in hot water.

Nourishing and Calming Tea (养血宁心茶)

Ingredients: 6g longan meat, 5g lily bulb, 3 pieces red dates, 3–6g wolfberry seeds

If you have difficulty falling asleep and feeling vexed, this tea may be able to help provided that the underlying syndrome is heart blood and yin deficiency. Longan meat and red dates nourish blood to calm the heart and mind for a sounder sleep. Lily bulb, which has a cool nature, can help to douse deficiency fire.

Preparation method: Infuse in hot water or boil the herbs for stronger concentration.

Longevity Tea (寿比南山茶)

Ingredients: 4–6g astragalus (*huangqi* 黄芪), 6g *huangjing* (黄精), 3–5g *zhigancao* (炙甘草), 3–6g wolfberry seeds

The two precious ingredients in this tea, *astragalus* and *huangjing*, help to enhance vital energy and longevity by tonifying qi and essence. *Huangjing* nourishes lung, spleen and kidney, helping to retard ageing. As pointed out in an earlier chapter, research has suggested that astragalus can help to slow down ageing by boosting the enzyme telomerase. *Zhigancao* is a mild qi tonic. As astragalus and *huangjing* are roots, they should be boiled for a stronger effect.

Preparation method: After boiling, cook with moderate heat for 30 to 40 minutes. Wolfberry seeds should be added in the last 15 minutes as it needs only a quick boil and can have a sour taste if it is cooked too long.

Digestion Tea (消食降脂茶)

Ingredients: 6g hawthorn, 4–6g *danshen* (丹参), 3–5g *zhigancao*, rock sugar (optional)

This tea assists in digesting a rich and heavy meal. It can be easily made by boiling three herbs with hawthorn berry as the main ingredient for promoting digestion of fats/lipids. *Danshen* plays a ministerial role by promoting blood flow and removing stasis. As hawthorn berry is sour, individuals who have weak stomachs should avoid this tea before meals. Pregnant women should drink this tea with caution as both hawthorn and danshen have the action of promoting blood flow. With its sweet flavour, *zhigancao* is added to mitigate the sourness of the tea. This tea can also be used in individuals who have mild coronary heart disease as clinical research suggests that both *danshen* and hawthorn may help to slow down atherosclerosis.

Preparation method: After boiling, cook for another 15–20 minutes.

Yin Nourishing and Thirst-Quenching Tea (养阴止渴茶)

Ingredients: 6g *dendobrium* (*shihu* 石斛), 3g *yuzhu* (玉竹), 4–5 slices American ginseng, 3–6g wolfberry seeds

This tea contains mainly yin tonics that promote the production of body fluids. It quenches thirst arising from yin deficiency, which can result in deficiency fire with thirst and dryness in the throat and mouth. Dendrobium and *yuzhu* help to nourish stomach and kidney yin and replenish fluids in the body. American ginseng not only nourishes yin but is also a qi tonic.

Preparation method: Steep the herbs in hot water or boil the herbs for a stronger concentration.

Guifei Complexion Tea (贵妃养颜茶)

Ingredients: 4g rose flowers, 2g jasmine flowers, 3–4 pieces red dates

A popular tea among the ladies, this fragrant flora tea helps to enhance one's complexion by promoting better qi and blood flow. With good flows in the body, there is sufficient blood to nourish and moisten the skin, bringing a healthy pink glow to the skin. Legend has it that the imperial concubine Yang Guifei of the Tang dynasty, who had a fabulously beautiful complexion, drank this tea regularly.

Preparation method: Infuse in hot water.

Chapter 15

The Prevention and Management
of Chronic Illnesses

To illustrate how TCM methods are applied to common chronic illnesses, we examine briefly its use in coronary heart disease, stroke, diabetes, and digestive disorders. These conditions have been chosen because TCM treatment in each case provides an interesting complement or alternative to Western medicine. The objective is to illustrate how TCM methods have been used in a clinical work and offer a comparison with biomedical methods.

15.1 Coronary Heart Disease

Coronary heart disease involves the narrowing of blood vessels supplying nutrients and oxygen to the heart. This narrowing is caused by dietary, genetic, ageing and lifestyle factors with build-up of plaque on arterial walls. Angina pain can occur when blood supply is inadequate.

TCM interprets coronary heart disease as an impediment to the free flow of qi and blood of the heart. The condition is classified under 'chest blockage with heart pain' (*xiongbi xintong* 胸痹心痛) and attributed to one or more of seven underlying syndromes, of which the most common are deficiency of heart qi and blood stasis.

In the absence of other syndromes associated with heart disease, the first syndrome of deficient heart qi is consistent with early or mild coronary heart disease. Blood stasis syndrome is usually found in more advanced stages of the disease when significant atherosclerosis has set in. Deficiency of heart qi usually occurs in the early stages, and the additional syndrome of blood stasis sets in as the disease progresses, hence we can regard qi deficiency as the root syndrome and blood stasis as the consequent syndrome of disease progression.

Deficiency of heart qi

Deficiency of heart qi is identified by symptoms of dull pain in the chest, heart palpitations, shortness of breath which worsens upon exertion, fatigue and sweating without exertion. The tongue is pale and slightly swollen, with tooth indentations and thin white fur; the pulse is slow, weak and thready or slow and irregular.

TCM treatment for the first syndrome consists of strengthening the body's qi level and promoting (regulating) its flow through qigong and taijiquan exercises, as well as diets containing foods and herbs that tonify qi, such as American ginseng, Chinese yam (*huaishan*), astragalus (*huangqi*), ginseng, and *dangshen*. A typical prescription formulation, appropriately modified to suit each patient's condition, would be *Baoyuan Tang* (保元汤) combined with *Ganmaidazao Tang* (甘麦大枣汤). The first uses ginseng and astragalus as the main components for boosting qi. The latter uses *xiaomai* (小麦) or wheat as the monarch herb to nourish heart yin and honey-baked liquorice (*zhigancao*) as the minister herb to promote flow along the heart meridian, invigorating the heart and tranquilising the mind.

Blood stasis

The syndrome of blood stasis has symptoms of stabbing pain or angina pain in the chest, sometimes spreading to the back and shoulders. It can be accompanied by prolonged "chest oppression" (胸闷), a TCM term for an uncomfortable depressive feeling of pressure on the chest. The tongue is dark with ecchymosis (bluish-black marks) and thin fur; pulse is wiry and astringent, or rapid and intermittent/irregular.

For the second syndrome, TCM treatment would typically encourage the consumption of foods and herbs that improve blood circulation and reduce blood stasis. These would include *danshen*, hawthorn (*shanzha*), red yeast rice (*hongqumi*), *chuanxiong*, safflower (*honghua*), peach kernel (*taoren*), black fungus, and tumeric.[35] In biomedical terms, these herbs are known to have mild vasodilating effects, rendering transient improved blood flow and symptomatic relief from angina pain. In the TCM framework, such vasodilating effects are only symptoms of more lasting changes brought about by 'resolving blood stasis', a claim which implies slower build-up of plaque and less impediment to blood flow. A typical prescription for blood stasis syndrome in the chest is the 'Decoction for Removing Blood Stasis in the Chest' (*Xuefu Zhuyu Tang* 血府逐瘀汤).

TCM as complementary treatment

Compared to Western treatments using various nitrates for vasodilation, blood thinners (like aspirin) to reduce the risk of blood clots, and surgical interventions like angioplasty and bypass surgery, TCM treatments are slower and cannot deal effectively with acute angina or emergency situations of coronary infarction. But they can be useful either as complementary treatment or, in mild cases, as an alternative to interventions like stenting.

TCM approaches to management of heart conditions using medicated diets and Chinese exercises can complement Western methods such as maintaining low cholesterol levels, exercises for cardiovascular fitness, and a diet rich in fibre and low in saturated and trans fats with generous amounts of fresh fruits and vegetables to promote endothelial health. The use of Chinese herbal supplements to improve qi and reduce blood stasis may be of significant help in

---

[35] Noted advocate of natural healing Dr Andrew Weil MD recommends the regular consumption of black fungus for coronary heart health. See Weil (1995) p166.

reducing arterial wall inflammation, hence contribute to the prevention and management of coronary heart disease.

15.2 Hypertension and Stroke

There are two major kinds of strokes, the ischaemic stroke and the haemorrhagic stroke.

Ischaemic stroke is by far the more common, being precipitated by sudden blocked blood flow in an artery of the brain. This could be caused by clotting at the artery (thrombosis). Or it could be a clot from another location, usually the heart or the carotid artery in the neck. The clot lodges itself within the artery (embolism), cutting off oxygen supply to part of the brain.

A haemorrhagic stroke results from rupture of an artery wall in the brain, leading to cerebral haemorrhage. It is commonly occurs with degenerative disease of the arteries and hypertension. The use of anticoagulants (blood thinners) like warfarin can also raise the risk of a haemorrhagic stroke.

Western medicine attributes strokes to risk factors like hypertension, smoking, excessive cholesterol (LDL) levels, and diabetes. Heart arrhythmia in the form of atrial fibrillation can also produce clots that travel to the brain.

Causes and treatment of stroke

TCM views the underlying conditions predisposing a person to strokes involve the endogenous wind pathogen (*feng* 风). Hence, the Chinese term for stroke is *zhong feng* (中风), or "attack by wind". Endogenous wind may arise from one or more of several syndromes, which include:

(a) weakness of yin and blood giving rise to liver heat and wind;
(b) overwork and strain stirring up liver wind;
(c) inappropriate diet that creates warm phlegm in the spleen, generating endogenous wind;

(d) emotional stress particularly anger triggering fire and the production of harmful wind.

One or more TCM syndromes may be observed with a stroke event. Which syndromes are observed depend on the kind of the stroke and the stage of progression, whether at the onset, in the immediate aftermath, or during the longer term recovery phase of the patient.

Chinese treatments directly address the prevailing syndromes at each stage of the evolution of the illness. In the early aftermath of a stroke, there is an emphasis on calming endogenous wind. In the later stages, the focus is on resolving phlegm and blood stasis. In the rehabilitation and recovery phase, this shifts to tonics for qi, blood and the yin of the liver and kidney.

At the onset and immediate aftermath stage, hyperactivity of liver yang, phlegm with wind, and stirring of liver wind (*ganfeng neidong* 肝风内动) are the common syndromes. *Tianma Gouteng Yin* (天麻钩藤饮), with variations to suit the patient, is most often used in the early stages.

At the later recovery stages, phlegm and blood stasis are often present, and the patient may suffer from severe qi deficiency and weakness of the liver and kidney. In these later stages, tonics with added ingredients for resolving blood stasis are used. An example is *Buyang Huanwu Tang* (补阳还五汤).

Stroke treatment usually combines herbal prescriptions, acupuncture and tuina, and is continually modified as the pathological state of the patient changes and new syndromes are exhibited.

Acupuncture for strokes

Acupuncture helps the rehabilitation process by enhancing flow of qi and blood in the body, leading to better recovery of motor skills and overall physiological functions by inducing beneficial changes in the blood flow to the brain. Common points used in post-stroke acupuncture treatment include *taichong* (太冲), *hegu* (合谷), *renzhong* (人中), *baihui* (百会), *sanyinjiao* (三阴交), *neiguan* (内关), *yanglingquan* (阳陵泉) and *quchi* (曲池). These acupoints can also be used in the treatment of hypertension. A fuller description of acupuncture points for stroke treatment is provided in chapter 12 on acupuncture.

Exercises

Exercises like qigong and taijiquan, for patients with sufficient mobility, are believed to enhance recovery from post-stroke disabilities. Chinese exercises work on improving blood and qi circulation, postural robustness and joint mobility, less on building muscular strength.

Social interaction within qigong groups may also help to improve patient morale and nurture the positive emotions that help recovery.

It would appear that a combination of Western and Chinese treatments can secure better results for the patient than a strict adherence to one regimen. When treatments are combined, attention must be paid to drug compatibility. For example, some Chinese herbs have mild anticoagulant properties that may over-enhance the effect of Western anticoagulant drugs.

15.3 Diabetes Mellitus

Diabetes mellitus is a disorder of carbohydrate metabolism in which sugars in the body are not oxidised to produce energy due to lack of insulin, leading to high blood glucose (sugar) level. It is one of the fastest-growing diseases in developed countries, some of which are witnessing epidemic-like growth in the disease.

There are two types of diabetes. Type 1 diabetes is an autoimmune disease in which the body's own immune system attacks the pancreas, leading to a decrease in insulin production. Type 2 diabetes is mainly a lifestyle disease attributable to poor dietary habits and an inactive lifestyle, with obesity, in particular waistline fat, as one of the major risk factors.

In type 2 diabetes, the body develops insulin resistance and is consequently unable to carry glucose into the body's cells either for storage or metabolism. In the longer run, insulin production drops and type 2 diabetes results.

The usual symptoms for both types of diabetes are thirst, hunger, weight loss, frequent urination, and lethargy.

TCM view of type 2 diabetes

There is no exact equivalent of diabetes in TCM. The symptoms associated with diabetes resemble closely a TCM condition recorded in the *Neijing* as *xiaoke* (消渴); *xiao* (消) means exhausting of the body's nutrients and *ke* (渴) means thirst. This term captures the classic symptoms of *xiaoke* as excessive thirst, frequent urination, hunger pangs, weight loss and sugar in the urine; these are similar to the typical symptoms of diabetes. It is less common but possible, however, for a patient to have the symptoms of *xiaoke* but blood tests do not show an abnormal sugar level. Conversely the patient can have high sugar level and not exhibit *xiaoke* symptoms. In modern TCM usage which has been influenced by biomedical terminology, the term *Tangniao Bing* (糖尿病) is commonly used to refer to diabetes and is not strictly differentiated from *xiaoke*.

TCM attributes *xiaoke* symptoms to yin deficiency, which is accompanied by "asthenic (deficiency) fire" and dryness (阴虚燥热). The illness can be categorised by dysfunctions of a particular organ and the TCM syndrome associated with it. All categories of the illness have in common symptoms of thirst, hunger and frequent urination to different degrees.

The *zang* organ which is affected in the early stage of *xiaoke* is the lung which has the underlying syndrome of lung heat with dryness (肺热津伤), also known as the upper trunk *xiaoke* (上消). The main symptom is thirst even after drinking, accompanied by excessive and frequent urination, dry tongue and mouth, vexatiousness, thin yellowish fur on the tongue with strong and fast pulse.

As the illness progresses, it affects the stomach and results in middle trunk *xiaoke* (中消) which can have two possible syndromes:

(i) Exuberance of stomach fire (胃热炽盛) which is characterized by hunger pangs, abnormally thin, constipation with dry stools and yellowish fur;

(ii) Deficiency in spleen qi and yin (气阴亏虚) which usually manifests in intense thirst, abnormally high appetite with loose stools, skinny, fatigue, light-red tongue with dry white fur and weak pulse.

The late stage of *xiaoke* usually damages kidney functions and results in lower trunk *xiaoke* (下消), with the syndrome of kidney yin deficiency (肾阴亏虚). The main symptoms are excessive and frequent urination, cloudy urine, dry lips, skinny, weak knees, soreness in the lower back, dry itchy skin, red tongue with little or no fur and a thready rapid pulse.

Treatment

The general TCM approach is to treat the syndromes that are presented rather than the disease directly. This may require replenishing yin, moisturising dryness and removing heat with the use of yin tonics.

In upper trunk *xiaoke,* the formulation used is modified *Xiaoke Fang* (消渴方) which nourishes yin and promotes the production of fluids to quench thirst. It also has ingredients to purge fire.

For middle trunk *xiaoke,* the typical formulation to address the exuberance of stomach fire syndrome is *Yunü Jian* (玉女煎) which nourishes yin and purges stomach fire. If there is deficiency in spleen qi and yin, the formulation is modified to *Qiweibaizhu San* (七味白术散) comprising mainly spleen-qi and yin tonics.

For lower trunk *xiaoke*, the formulation commonly used is *Liuweidihuang Wan* (六味地黄丸), a classical yin tonic for the kidney and liver.

Blood stasis syndrome may be seen in late-stage diabetic patients with complications such as nephropathy, retinopathy, and chronic heart disease. Herbs with blood promoting and stasis removing actions are added to the formulation.

Recent research suggests that some herbs in TCM may be helpful in the control and management of blood glucose level. These include *huangqi*, purslane (*machixian* 马齿苋), *shanzhuyu* and *rougui*.

15.4 Digestive Disorders

The legendary physician Li Dongyuan (李东垣) of the Jin-Yuan dynasties focused on care of the digestive system for health and longevity, and postulated that damage to the spleen and stomach was the root cause of most illnesses.

The TCM spleen governs the processing and transforming food into nutrients that feed other organs and the rest of the body, pairing with the stomach in its work. The spleen nourishes the body and replenishes the store of qi, blood and essence or *jing* in the vital organs. By providing nutrients to the kidney to replenish the store of qi and *jing*, the spleen serves as the foundation of postnatal health.

Spleen functions are inhibited by dampness, characterised by "stickiness" that impedes the flow of qi, resulting in qi stagnation in the abdomen. If not treated, weak qi and/or qi stagnation exacerbates dampness which progresses to the accumulation of phlegm. Improper diet such as oily and fried foods, and brooding accompanied by anxiety, are the leading causal factors for damage of spleen functions. The result is gastrointestinal disorders such as poor appetite, a bloated abdomen, wind, and loose stools. It can also lead to the irritable bowel syndrome. The high incidence of digestive disorders in high-stress societies like Beijing, New York and Singapore may well be associated with stressful lifestyles that harm the spleen.

Herbal supplements used to strengthen spleen functions include dried tangerine peels (*chenpi*), *sharen* and *banxia* which can smoothen the flow of spleen qi and resolve dampness and phlegm. *Dangshen, shanyao, huangqi* and red dates are used to tonify spleen qi. These herbs can be used as ingredients for spleen-healthy meals, although *sharen* and *banxia* are not so tasty and tend to be used more in medical prescriptions. A delicious nourishing rice porridge with *huangqi*, red dates and Chinese yam can be used to maintain healthy functioning of the spleen and stomach.

Common formulations for spleen disorders include *Sijunzi Tang, Shenling Baizhu San*, and *Xiangsha Liujunzi Tang*.[36] These formulations combine qi tonics with qi regulation herbs to remove dampness and restore qi flow.

Irritable Bowel Syndrome (IBS)

The Irritable Bowel Syndrome (*Changyiji Zonghezheng* 肠易激综合征) is a recurrent condition with abdominal pain and constipation and/or diarrhoea, often with bloating of the abdomen and dyspepsia. There is no detectable structural disease. It can continue for years. The condition is often associated with stress or anxiety and may follow an episode of intestinal infection. In Western medicine, the cause is idiopathic (not known).[37]

TCM regards IBS as a condition associated with imbalances and/or stagnation in the spleen. It is not a disease in its own right, but one of several manifestations of imbalance and qi stagnation in the spleen. This could take the form of dampness in the spleen when spleen qi is weak or does not flow properly, the result of improper diet or exposure to the dampness pathogen. It can also be the

---

[36] See Chapter 7 and Annex 2 for these formulations.
[37] Oxford (2007).

consequence of an "exuberant" liver over-restraining the spleen, a condition that we explained with the five element model in an chapter 4 of this book. The exuberant liver is usually the result of stress and anxiety, causing stagnation in liver qi flow and progressing to liver fire.

IBS is frequently encountered in TCM practice especially among city dwellers in high-stress environments. Stress harms the liver, stoking exuberance and fire. Also, consumption of fried and high-fat foods makes for a veritable breeding ground for spleen dampness.

TCM treatment for IBS comprises mainly resolving spleen dampness with herbs and formulations like *Xiangsha Liujunzi Tang* or calming the liver with *Xiaoyao San*, of course with variations customised to the other syndromes of the patient.[38] IBS-like conditions are frequently encountered in TCM clinical work and there is considerable clinical evidence of the efficacy of TCM treatments.

Conclusion

In all the four cases above, TCM provides both complementary and alternative treatments to common chronic illnesses, working largely from the vantage point of restoring imbalances in the body system and encouraging the body's own healing powers to ameliorate symptoms or bring about recovery. It is patient-centric in the sense of addressing directly the nature of the underlying syndromes present and adapting to changing syndromes as the illness evolves and progresses in each patient.

Despite its ancient origins, TCM has shown remarkable resilience in preserving a healthcare role in modern scientific societies.

---

[38] See Annex 2 and Chapter 7.

Chapter 16

The Future of Chinese Medicine

Even as TCM clinics and colleges flourish in East Asia and many Western countries in the 21st century, doubts about its scientific credentials persist among biomedical scientists nurtured in the reductionism of molecular and cellular biology and statistical methods in evidence-based medicine.

Nevertheless, TCM continues to play a significant role in healthcare worldwide. Among its followers, it enjoys a reputation for healing no less than that of biomedicine. However, the lack of understanding of TCM concepts and methods remains a barrier to its appreciation by biomedical scientists and Western doctors and hinders even the more familiar and proven parts of TCM from being incorporated into mainstream medicine.

Ironically, several Western countries have in a sense gone further in recognising TCM than health regulatory authorities in some East Asian countries that already have a long tradition in Chinese medicine. In the United States, for example, acupuncture is offered by state-licensed practitioners and eligible for insurance claims. The TCM department at the reputable Cleveland Clinic offers herbal and acupuncture treatments despite acknowledging that many of the therapies lack sufficient evidence of the kind accepted by modern medicine. But the clinic seems to recognize that the continued demand for such treatment by patients may eventually be vindicated by rigorous clinical studies. In contrast, in the former British territories Hong Kong and Singapore, a strict separation is kept between TCM and Western medicine, with TCM enjoying generous support from charitable institutions, but little state support.

Evidence-based medicine

One of the beliefs common among Western medical practitioners is that Western medicine is evidence-based whilst TCM is not. This is at best a half truth, at worst a biased stance against a competing school of medicine.

Much revolves around what counts as evidence-based medicine. Advances in statistical inference techniques led to the popularity of double-blind randomized controlled trials (RCTs) in the middle of the 20th century. Big pharmaceutical companies have dominated the drug industry by advocating large-scale RCTs as the gold standard. As these trials are notoriously costly to run (US$1 billion being not an unusual figure for a new drug), only these "big pharmas" can afford them. These pharmaceutical giants also have the resources to secure and defend intellectual property rights and market the successful drugs to recover research and development and clinical trial costs. Hence new drug discovery became virtually the preserve of Big Pharmas who totally dominate the industry.

TCM herbs and formulations face formidable difficulties to qualify as therapeutic drugs under such regulatory regimes. To begin with, TCM clinical trials are technically much more difficult to run because of the higher complexity with TCM therapy. For example, the drugs should be syndrome-targeted in TCM practice. A disease like diabetes or ischaemic heart disease has several possible syndrome combinations requiring different treatments, greatly complicating the protocols for RCTs.

From a business point of view, it is almost impossible to get funding for large-scale clinical trials for TCM formulations as nearly all of them have been around for centuries, and there are no patents for them. Hence there is no profit motive for drug companies to conduct the trials. In principle only state health institutions or philanthropists would finance such trials. In practice few if any do so.

Is there a way forward for the validation of TCM medications?

Looking at the history of modern medicine, we find that many of its most important advances preceded the advent of double-blind RCTs in the early 1960s. These include the discovery of vaccines, viruses and bacteria as proximate causes of disease, and penicillin and other antibiotics. Observational studies using clinical data collated and analysed to minimize selection bias, as well as carefully recorded case studies, all helped to bring about these great discoveries.

The overemphasis on RCTs as the gold standard for clinical trials has been criticized by philosophers of science and medicine as well as respected biomedical scientists. The prominent British philosopher John Worrall, mindful of RCTs being only a recent invention, puts it pointedly, "What on earth was medicine based on before?"[39]

Sir Michael Rawlins, former chairman of the National Institute for Clinical Excellence (NICE), an expert body on clinical trials, opines:

> The notion that evidence can be reliably placed in hierarchies is illusory. Hierarchies place RCTs on an undeserved pedestal ... Although the technique has advantages it also has significant disadvantages. Observational studies too have defects, but they also have merit. Decision makers need to assess and appraise all the available evidence irrespective as to whether it has been derived from RCTs or observational studies.[40]

A case can be made for TCM formulations to given greater credence based on observational studies, case studies, and smaller-scale clinical trials. The patient-centric nature of TCM prescribes individualised treatment against mass uniform treatment with the

---

[39] Worrall (2002)
[40] Rawlins (2008)

same formulation and dosage regardless of different underlying syndromes. This makes it difficult to conduct RCTs, and it is more realistic to use observational studies employing reliable patient data from TCM clinics.[41]

Modern medicine and its discontents

In his insightful work *The Rise and Fall of Modern Medicine*, British physician and medical writer James Le Fanu points out a puzzling paradox. Despite quantum leaps in medical science over the last seventy years since the discovery of the structure of the DNA and dazzling advances in molecular biology, we have failed to answer some basic questions in medical science. Le Fanu laments, "Reductionism, the explanation of the phenomena of disease at the most fundamental level of the gene and its products, fails to explain the fact that causes of common diseases are either age-determined or biological and for the most part unknown. Medicine's post-war success, built on the chance discovery of drugs and technological innovation, concealed the fact that its impressive achievements had been won without the necessity to understand the nature or causation of disease. And now medicine still knows the cause of only a fraction of the diseases in the textbooks."[42]

Among the diseases of unknown cause are multiple sclerosis, rheumatoid arthritis, schizophrenia, and most forms of cancer.

The idea that most diseases are idiopathic, or of unknown origin, is valid only if we think that only reductionist explanations make sense, that is, reducing causation to viruses, bacteria, and cellular abnormalities. TCM provides alternative explanations using holistic models, interpreting human physiology using its own sets of concepts like qi, meridians and organs. Diseases are caused by

---

[41] See Hong (2016) Chapter 8 for a more detailed treatment of this subject.

[42] Le Fanu (2011). The quotation has been combined with extracts from several passages to read more smoothly.

imbalances and disturbed flows in the body, themselves mostly the result of poor living habits as well as environmental and emotional stress. The *Huangdi Neijing* argues that modern man changed his lifestyle and diet, which over many millennia had been adapted to man's natural environment, as the most basic cause of illness. This holds true even more today than it did two thousand years ago.

There is hope in the new science of systems biology. This focuses on interactions within biological systems and is more holistic than reductionist. Its principal aim is to model cells and tissues functioning as a system with complex internal networks. This new dimension of biomedical science may hold promise for a degree of convergence between biomedicine and TCM.[43]

Conclusions

We hope that with a better understanding of the scientific basis for Chinese medicine and more open minds, there will eventually be a better appreciation of TCM as an alternative system of healing and explaining illness. At the same time, the TCM scientific community must press on with ever more rigorous clinical testing of TCM interventions.

Mainstream medicine should not be just Western medicine. It should be evidence-based medicine. But we should take a more liberal view of what evidence we accept, be it for TCM or Western interventions.

---

[43] Hong (2017)

Annex 1

Common Chinese Herbs

	Diaphoretic Herbs with Pungent Warm Property 辛温解表药		
Name of Herb	Flavour and Nature	Meridian Tropism	Actions
Mahuang 麻黄 (Ephedra)	Pungent and slightly bitter; Warm	Lung and bladder	1. Induce sweating to relieve superficies 2. Ventilate the lung to relieve asthma 3. Promote diuresis
Guizhi 桂枝 (Cinnamon)	Pungent and sweet; Warm	Heart, lung and bladder	1. Induce sweating to relieve superficies 2. Reinforce yang and warm the meridians
Fangfeng 防风 (Divaricate Saposhnikovia Root)	Pungent and sweet; Slightly warm	Bladder, liver and spleen	1. Expel wind 2. Resolve dampness to relieve pain 3. Relieve spasms
Shengjiang 生姜 (Fresh Ginger)	Pungent; Warm	Lung, spleen and stomach	1. Expel wind-cold pathogens 2. Warm the abdomen to relieve nausea and vomiting 3. Warm the lung to relieve cough
Xinyi 辛夷 (Magnolia Biondii Flower)	Pungent; Warm	Lung and stomach	1. Expel wind-cold pathogen 2. Clear the nasal passageway

(Continued)

(Continued)

Name of Herb	Flavour and Nature	Meridian Tropism	Actions
Diaphoretic Herbs with Pungent Cool Property 辛凉解表药			
Cang'erzi 苍耳子 (Siberian Cocklebur Fruit)	Pungent and bitter; Warm; Slightly toxic	Lung	1. Expel wind-cold pathogen 2. Clear the nasal passageway 3. Dispel wind-dampness 4. Relieve pain
Chaihu 柴胡 (Chinese Thorowax Root)	Pungent and bitter; Slightly cold	Liver and gall bladder	1. Relieve exterior syndrome 2. Anti-pyretic 3. Regulate stagnation of liver-qi 4. Uplift yang-qi
Juhua 菊花 (Chrysanthemum flower)	Pungent, bitter and sweet; Slightly cold	Lung and liver	1. Expel wind-heat 2. Clear liver heat to improve vision 3. Calm and suppress liver-yang 4. Eliminate toxins
Sangye 桑叶 (Mulberry Leaf)	Sweet and bitter; Cold	Lung and liver	1. Expel wind-heat 2. Clear lung-heat and nourish dryness 3. Calm and suppress liver-yang 4. Clear liver-heat to improve vision
Bohe 薄荷 (Peppermint Leaf)	Pungent; Cool	Lung and liver	1. Expel wind-heat from the head, eye and throat 2. Soothe liver and regulate liver-qi stagnation
Gegen 葛根 (Kudzuvine Root)	Pungent and sweet; Cool	Spleen and stomach	1. Anti-pyretic 2. Promote production of fluids to quench thirst 3. Uplift yang-qi to stop diarrhoea 4. Promote the outburst of measles

Herbs for Clearing Heat and Purging Fire 清熱瀉火药

Name of Herb	Flavour and Nature	Meridian Tropism	Actions
Shigao 石膏 (Gypsum)	Sweet and pungent; Very cold	Lung and stomach	Raw form 1. Clear heat and purge fire 2. Remove vexation and quench thirst Calcinated form: Stop bleeding and promote the growth of tissue (for treating ulcers)
Zhimu 知母 (Anemarrhena Rhizome)	Bitter and sweet; Cold	Lung, stomach and kidney	1. Clear heat and purge fire 2. Promote the production of fluids for moistening
Danzhuye 淡竹叶 (Lophatherum Herb)	Sweet and bland; Cold	Heart, stomach and small intestine	1. Clear heat and purge fire 2. Relieve vexation 3. Promote diuresis
Zhizi 栀子 (Cape Jasmine Fruit)	Bitter; Cold	Heart, lung and triple energiser	1. Purge fire to remove vexation 2. Clear heat-dampness 3. Cool the blood and eliminate toxins. Charred form can stop bleeding
Xiakucao 夏枯草 (Common Selfheal Fruit-Spike)	Pungent and bitter; Cold	Liver and gall bladder	1. Clear heart and purge fire to improve vision 2. Disperse abnormal growth/masses to reduce swelling
Juemingzi 决明子 (Cassia Seeds)	Sweet, bitter and salty; Slightly cold	Liver and large intestine	1. Clear liver-heat to improve vision 2. Moisten the large intestine to promote bowel movement

(Continued)

Herbs for Clearing Heat-Dampness 清热燥湿药			
Name of Herb	Flavour and Nature	Meridian Tropism	Actions
Huangqin 黄芩 (Baical Skullcap Root/*Radix Scutellariae*)	Bitter; Cold	Lung, gall bladder, spleen, stomach, large and small intestine	1. Clear heat and dry dampness 2. Purge fire and eliminate toxins 3. Stop bleeding 4. Prevent miscarriage
Kushen 苦参 (Light-yellow Sophora Root)	Bitter; Cold	Heart, liver, stomach, large intestine and bladder	1. Clear heat and dry dampness 2. Kill parasites, fungus 3. Promote diuresis

Herbs for Clearing Heat and Eliminating Toxins 清热解毒药			
Name of Herb	Flavour and Nature	Meridian Tropism	Actions
Jinyinhua 金银花 (Honeysuckle Flower)	Sweet; Cold	Lung, heart and stomach	1. Eliminate heat and toxins 2. Expel wind-heat pathogens
Lianqiao 连翘 (Weeping Forsythia Capsule)	Bitter; Slightly cold	Lung, heart and small intestine	1. Eliminate heat and toxins 2. Disperse masses/abnormal growth to reduce swelling 3. Expel wind-heat pathogens
Chuanxinlian 穿心莲 (Common Andrographis Herb)	Bitter; Cold	Lung, heart, large intestine and bladder	1. Eliminate heat and toxins 2. Cool the blood 3. Reduce swelling 4. Resolve dampness

Herbs for Clearing Heat and Eliminating Toxins 清热解毒药			
Name of Herb	**Flavour and Nature**	**Meridian Tropism**	**Actions**
Banlangen 板蓝根 (Isatis root)	Bitter; Cold	Heart and stomach	1. Eliminate heat and toxins 2. Cool the blood 3. Soothe the throat
Yuxingcao 鱼腥草 (Heartleaf Houttuynia)	Pungent; Slightly cold	Lung	1. Eliminate heat and toxins 2. Reduce abscess by promoting pus discharge 3. Remove dampness by promoting diuresis
Machixian 马齿苋 (Purslane)	Sour; Cold	Liver and large intestine	1. Eliminate heat and toxins 2. Cool the blood to stop bleeding 3. Stop dysentry
Pugongyin 蒲公英 (Dandelion)	Bitter and sweet; Cold	Liver and stomach	1. Eliminate heat and toxins 2. Disperse abnormal growth/masses to reduce swelling 3. Promote diuresis
Banbianlian 半边莲	Pungent; Neutral	Heart, lung and small intestine	1. Eliminate heat and toxins 2. Promote diuresis to relieve edema
Baihua Sheshecao 白花蛇舌草 (Oldenlandia)	Sweet and slightly bitter; Cold	Stomach, large and small intestine	1. Eliminate heat and toxins 2. Remove dampness by promoting diuresis

(*Continued*)

Heat-Clearing and Blood-Cooling Herbs 清热凉血药

Name of Herb	Flavour and Nature	Meridian Tropism	Actions
Xuanshen 玄参 (Figwort Root)	Sweet, salty and bitter; Slightly cold	Lung, stomach and kidney	1. Clear heat and cool the blood 2. Purge fire and remove toxins 3. Nourish yin
Mudanpi 牡丹皮 (Tree Peony Root)	Bitter and sweet; Slightly cold	Heart, liver and kidney	1. Clear heat and cool the blood 2. Promote blood flow and remove stasis
Shengdihuang 生地黄 (Raw Rehmannia Root)	Sweet and bitter; Cold	Heart, liver and kidney	1. Clear heat and cool the blood 2. Nourish yin and promote the production of fluids

Herbs for Clearing Asthenic Heat 清虚热药

Name of Herb	Flavour and Nature	Meridian Tropism	Actions
Qinghao 青蒿 (Sweet wormwood)	Bitter and pungent; Cold	Liver and gall bladder	1. Clear asthenic heat and summer heat 2. Cool the blood 3. Treat malaria

Purgatives 泻下药			
Name of Herb	Flavour and Nature	Meridian Tropism	Actions
Dahuang 大黄 (Rhubarb)	Bitter; Cold	Spleen, stomach, large intestine, liver and pericardium	1. Promote bowel movement by clearing heat and purging fire 2. Cool blood and remove toxins 3. Remove blood stasis
Fanxieye 番泻叶 (Senna Leaf)	Sweet and bitter; Cold	Large intestine	Purge to promote bowel movement
Huomaren 火麻仁 (Hemp Seed)	Sweet; Neutral	Spleen, stomach and large intestine	Promote bowel movement by moistening the intestine

(*Continued*)

	Herbs for Resolving Dampness 化湿药		
Name of Herb	Flavour and Nature	Meridian Tropism	Actions
Huoxiang 藿香 (Cablin Patchouli Herb)	Pungent; Slightly warm	Spleen, stomach and lung	1. Resolve dampness 2. Relieve nausea and vomiting 3. Clear summer-heat
Cangzhu 苍术 (Atractylodes Rhizome)	Pungent and bitter; Warm	Spleen, stomach and liver	1. Dry dampness and strengthen the spleen 2. Expel wind and disperse the cold
Houpo 厚朴 (Officinal Magnolia Bark)	Pungent and bitter; Warm	Spleen, stomach, lung and large intestine	1. Dry dampness and resolve phlegm 2. Promote the descent of qi to remove stagnation
Sharen 砂仁 (Villous Amomum Fruit)	Pungent; Warm	Spleen, stomach and kidney	1. Resolve dampness and regulate qi 2. Warm the abdomen and stop diarrhoea 3. Prevent miscarriage
Baidoukou 白豆蔻 (White Cardamon Fruit)	Pungent; Warm	Spleen, stomach and lung	1. Resolve dampness and regulate qi 2. Warm the abdomen to relieve nausea and vomiting

Herbs for Removing Wind-Dampness 祛风湿药			
Name of Herb	**Flavour and Nature**	**Meridian Tropism**	**Actions**
Wujiapi 五加皮 (Slenderstyle Acanthopanax Bark)	Pungent and bitter; Warm	Liver and kidney	1. Remove wind-dampness 2. Tonify the liver and kidney 3. Strengthen the ligaments and bone 4. Promote diuresis

Diuretics 利水渗湿药			
Name of Herb	**Flavour and Nature**	**Meridian Tropism**	**Actions**
Fuling 茯苓 (Poria)	Sweet and bland; Neutral	Heart, spleen and kidney	1. Promote diuresis to drain dampness and relieve edema 2. Invigorate spleen 3. Tranquilise the mind
Yiyiren 薏苡仁 (Job's Tears)	Sweet and bland; Cool	Spleen, stomach and lung	1. Promote diuresis to drain dampness and relieve edema 2. Invigorate spleen 3. Relieve joint pain 4. Clear heat and promote pus discharge
Dongguaren 冬瓜仁 (Winter melon seeds)	Sweet; Cool	Spleen and small intestine	1. Clear lung-heat and resolve phlegm 2. Remove dampness and promote pus discharge

(Continued)

Herbs for Regulating *Qi* 理气药

Name of Herb	Flavour and Nature	Meridian Tropism	Actions
Chenpi 陈皮 (Dried tangerine peel)	Pungent and bitter; Warm	Spleen and lung	1. Regulate qi and invigorate spleen 2. Dry dampness and resolve phlegm
Xiangfu 香附 (Nutgrass Galingale Rhizome)	Pungent, slightly bitter and sweet; Neutral	Liver, spleen and triple energiser	1. Regulate liver-qi stagnation 2. Regulate menstruation and relieve pain 3. Regulate spleen and stomach-qi
Meiguihua 玫瑰花 (Rose flower)	Sweet and slightly bitter; Warm	Spleen and liver	1. Regulate liver-qi stagnation 2. Promote blood flow to relieve pain

Herbs for Promoting Digestion 消食药

Name of Herb	Flavour and Nature	Meridian Tropism	Actions
Shanzha 山楂 (Hawthorn)	Sweet and sour; Slightly warm	Spleen, stomach and liver	1. Promote digestion 2. Regulate qi and remove stasis
Maiya 麦芽 (Germinated Barley)	Sweet; Neutral	Spleen, stomach and liver	1. Promote digestion and strengthen the stomach 2. Relieve breast engorgement. Stop lactation.
Laifuzi 莱菔子 (Radish seed)	Sweet and pungent; Neutral	Spleen, stomach and lung	1. Promote digestion and relieve abdomen distension 2. Promote the descent of qi and resolve dampness

Interior Warming Herbs 温里药

Name of Herb	Flavour and Nature	Meridian Tropism	Actions
Fuzi 附子 (Lateralis Preparata)	Pungent and sweet; Very Hot; Toxic	Heart, spleen and kidney	1. Restore yang (for severe deficiency of yang) 2. Strengthen yang by restoring fire 3. Disperse cold to alleviate pain
Ganjiang 干姜 (Zingiber Dried Ginger)	Pungent; Hot	Spleen, stomach, kidney, heart and lung	1. Warm the abdomen and disperse cold 2. Restore yang to warm and clear the collaterals 3. Warm the lung to resolve rheum
Rougui 肉桂 (Cassia Bark)	Pungent and sweet; Very Hot	Kidney, spleen, heart and liver	1. Strengthen yang by restoring fire 2. Disperse cold to alleviate pain 3. Warm the meridians to clear the collaterals 4. Return fire to the origin (kidney)
Huajiao 花椒 (Pricklyash Peel)	Pungent; Warm	Spleen, stomach and kidney	1. Warm the abdomen to relieve pain 2. Kill parasites to relieve itching

Hemostatics 止血药

Name of Herb	Flavour and Nature	Meridian Tropism	Actions
Sanqi 三七 (Panax notoginseng)	Sweet and slightly bitter; Warm	Liver and stomach	1. Remove blood stasis to stop bleeding 2. Promote blood circulation to relieve pain

(Continued)

Herbs for Promoting Blood Circulation and Removing Stasis 活血化瘀药

Name of Herb	Flavour and Nature	Meridian Tropism	Actions
Chuanxiong 川芎 (Sichuan Lovage Rhizome)	Pungent; Warm	Liver, gall bladder and pericardium	1. Promote blood circulation and regulate qi 2. Expel wind to relieve pain
Jianghuang 姜黄 (Tumeric)	Pungent and bitter; Warm	Spleen and liver	1. Promote blood circulation and regulate qi 2. Clear the collaterals to relieve pain
Moyao 没药 (Myrrh)	Pungent and bitter; Neutral	Heart, liver and spleen	1. Promote blood circulation to relieve pain 2. Reduce swelling and promote healing
Danshen 丹参 (Red Sage Root)	Bitter; Slightly cold	Heart, pericardium, and liver	1. Promote blood circulation to regulate menstruation 2. Remove stasis to relieve pain 3. Cool the blood to promote the healing of carbuncle 4. Remove vexation and calm the mind
Taoren 桃仁 (Peach Seed)	Bitter and sweet; Neutral; Slightly toxic	Heart, liver and large intestine	1. Promote blood circulation and remove stasis 2. Moisten the large intestine to promote bowel movement 3. Relieve cough and dyspnea
Honghua 红花 (Safflower)	Pungent; Warm	Heart and liver	1. Promote blood circulation and menstruation 2. Remove blood stasis to relieve pain

Herbs for Resolving Phlegm and Relieving Cough and Dyspnea 止咳化痰平喘药

Name of Herb	Flavour and Nature	Meridian Tropism	Actions
Banxia 半夏 (Pinellia Tuber)	Pungent; Warm; Toxic	Spleen, stomach and lung	1. Dry dampness and resolve phlegm 2. Relieve nausea and vomiting by suppressing the adverse rise of qi 3. Relieve abdominal distension and disperse masses
Jiegeng 桔梗 (Hogfennel Root)	Bitter and pungent; Neutral	Lung	1. Disperse lung-qi 2. Expel phlegm 3. Soothe the throat 4. Promote the discharge of pus
Gualou 瓜蒌 (Snakegourd Fruit)	Sweet and slightly bitter; Cold	Lung, stomach and large intestine	1. Clear heat and resolve phlegm 2. Regulate qi stagnation in the chest and disperse abnormal masses/growths 3. Moisten the large intestine to promote bowel movement
Chuanbeimu 川贝母 (Tendrilleaf Fritillary Bulb)	Bitter and Sweet; Slightly cold	Lung and heart	1. Clear heat and resolve phlegm 2. Moisten the lung to relieve cough 3. Disperse abnormal masses or growths to reduce swelling
Zhebeimu 浙贝母 (Thunberg Fritillary Bulb)	Bitter; Cold	Lung and heart	1. Clear heat and resolve phlegm 2. Disperse abnormal masses or growths to promote healing of carbuncle

(*Continued*)

(Continued)

Herbs for Resolving Phlegm and Relieving Cough and Dyspnea 止咳化痰平喘药			
Name of Herb	Flavour and Nature	Meridian Tropism	Actions
Luohanguo 罗汉果 (Monk Fruit)	Sweet; Cool	Lung and large intestine	1. Clear heat from the lung and soothe the throat 2. Resolve phlegm and relieve cough 3. Moisten the large intestine to promote bowel movement
Kuxingren 苦杏仁 (Bitter Apricot Seed)	Bitter; Slightly warm; Slightly toxic	Lung and large intestine	1. Relieve cough and dyspnea 2. Moisten the large intestine to promote bowel movement
Ziyuan 紫苑 (Tatarian Aster Root)	Bitter, sweet and pungent; Slightly warm	Lung	1. Moisten the lung and resolve phlegm to relieve cough
Kuandonghua 款冬花 (Common Clotsfoot Flower)	Pungent and slightly bitter; Warm	Lung	1. Moisten the lung, promote the descending of lung-qi and resolve phlegm to relieve cough
Pipaye 枇杷叶 (Loquat Leaf)	Bitter; Slightly cold	Lung and stomach	1. Clear lung heat to relieve cough 2. Promote the descent of qi to relieve nausea and vomiting
Baiguo 白果 (Ginkgo Seed)	Sweet, bitter and astringent; Neutral; Toxic	Lung	1. Astringe lung and resolve phlegm to relieve dyspnea 2. Stop abnormal vagina discharge (leucorrhoea) and reduce urination

Calmatives 安神药

Name of Herb	Flavour and Nature	Meridian Tropism	Actions
Longgu 龙骨 (Dragon Bone)	Sweet and astringent; Neutral	Heart, lung and kidney	1. Tranquilise the mind 2. Calm the liver to suppress liver-yang 3. Arrest fluids (calcinated form)
Suanzaoren 酸枣仁 (Spine Date Seed)	Sour and sweet; Neutral	Heart, liver and gall bladder	1. Nourish the heart and liver 2. Calm the mind 3. Arrest sweating
Yejiaoteng 夜交藤	Sweet; Neutral	Heart and liver	1. Nourish the blood to calm the mind 2. Expel wind to clear the collaterals
Baiziren 柏子仁 (Chinese Arborvitae Kernel)	Sweet; Neutral	Heart, kidney and large intestine	1. Nourish the heart to calm the mind 2. Moisten the intestine to promote bowel movement
Hehuanpi 合欢皮 (Silktree Albizia Bark)	Sweet; Neutral	Heart, liver and lung	1. Alleviate depression to calm the mind 2. Promote blood circulation to relieve swelling
Lingzhi 灵芝 (Lucid Ganoderma)	Sweet; Neutral	Heart, lung, liver and kidney	1. Strengthen qi to calm the mind 2. Relieve cough and asthma

(Continued)

Qi Tonics 补气药

Name of Herb	Flavour and Nature	Meridian Tropism	Actions
Renshen 人参 (Ginseng)	Sweet, Slightly bitter; Neutral	Lung, spleen and heart	1. Invigorate qi 2. Tonify the spleen and strengthen the lung 3. Promote the production of fluids 4. Calm the nerves for better concentration and also sounder sleep
Xiyangshen 西洋参 (American Ginseng)	Sweet, Slightly bitter; Cool	Lung, heart, kidney and spleen	1. Invigorate qi and nourish yin 2. Clear heat and promote the production of fluids
Dangshen 党参 (Codonopsis Root)	Sweet; Neutral	Spleen and lung	1. Invigorate the spleen and lung functions by tonifying their qi 2. Tonify blood 3. Promote the production of fluids
Taizishen 太子参 (Heterophylly Falsesatarwort Root)	Sweet, Slightly bitter; Neutral	Spleen and lung	1. Invigorate qi and strengthen the spleen functions 2. Promote the production of fluids to moisten the lung
Huangqi 黄芪 (Astragalus)	Sweet; Slightly warm	Spleen and lung	1. Strengthen the spleen functions 2. Uplift yang-qi 3. Consolidate the exterior to strengthen the body's defence against external pathogens 4. Promote diuresis and the healing of wounds/ulcers

Qi Tonics 补气药

Name of Herb	Flavour and Nature	Meridian Tropism	Actions
Baizhu 白术 (Largehead Astractylodes Rhizome)	Sweet and bitter; Warm	Spleen and stomach	1. Strengthen spleen and tonify qi 2. Dry dampness and promote diuresis 3. Stop perspiration 4. Prevent miscarriage
Shanyao 山药 (Chinese Yam)	Sweet; Neutral	Spleen, lung and kidney	1. Tonify the spleen and nourish the stomach 2. Promote the production of fluids and tonify the lung 3. Tonify the kidney 4. Conserve essence
Gancao 甘草 (Liquorice Root)	Sweet; Neutral	Heart, lung, spleen and stomach	1. Tonify the spleen 2. Resolve phlegm and relieve cough 3. Relieve pain 4. Clear heat and eliminate toxins (raw liquorice) 5. Regulate the actions of herbs in a prescription
Dazao 大枣 (Chinese Date)	Sweet; Warm	Spleen, stomach and heart	1. Strengthen the spleen functions and tonify qi 2. Nourish blood to calm the mind
Baibiandou 白扁豆 (White Hyacinth Bean)	Sweet; Slightly Warm	Spleen and stomach	1. Tonify the spleen 2. Resolve dampness

(Continued)

Yang Tonics 补阳药

Name of Herb	Flavour and Nature	Meridian Tropism	Actions
Lurong 鹿茸 (Hairy Antler)	Sweet and salty; Warm	Kidney and lung liver	1. Tonify kidney-yang 2. Tonify blood and essence 3. Strengthen the bone and tendons 4. Regulate the *chong* 冲 and *ren* 任 vessels (they govern the menstruation) 5. Promote the healing of sores/ulcers
Yinyanghuo 淫羊藿 (Horny-goat Weed)	Pungent and sweet; Warm	Kidney and liver	1. Tonify the kidney and boost yang 2. Expel wind and remove dampness
Duzhong 杜仲 (Eucommia Bark)	Sweet; Warm	Liver and kidney	1. Tonify the kidney and liver 2. Strengthen the bones and tendons 3. Prevent miscarriage
Dongchongxiacao 冬虫夏草 (Cordyceps)	Sweet and salty; Warm	Kidney and lung	1. Tonify the kidney and lung 2. Resolve phlegm 3. Stop bleeding
Hetaoren 核桃仁 (Walnut)	Sweet; Warm	Kidney, lung and large intestine	1. Tonify the kidney and warm the lung 2. Moisten the large intestine to promote bowel movement

Blood Tonics 补血药

Name of Herb	Flavour and Nature	Meridian Tropism	Actions
Shudihuang 熟地黄 (Processed Rehmannia Root)	Sweet; Slightly warm	Liver and kidney	1. Tonify blood and nourish yin 2. Supplement essence and marrow
Ejiao 阿胶	Sweet; Neutral	Lung, liver and kidney	1. Tonify blood and nourish yin 2. Moisten the lung 3. Stop bleeding
Heshouwu 何首乌 (Root of Tuber Fleeceflower)	Bitter, sweet, astringent; Slightly warm	Kidney and liver	Processed form: 1. Tonify and enrich blood Raw form: 1. Eliminate toxins 2. Treat malaria 3. Moisten the large intestine to promote bowel movement
Longyanrou 龙眼肉 (Longan Meat)	Sweet; Warm	Heart and spleen	1. Tonify the heart and spleen 2. Nourish blood to calm the mind
Danggui 当归 (Chinese Angelica)	Sweet and pungent; Warm	Liver, heart and spleen	1. Tonify blood and regulate menstruation 2. Promote blood circulation to relieve pain 3. Moisten the large intestine to promote bowel movement

(Continued)

Yin Tonics 补阴药

Name of Herb	Flavour and Nature	Meridian Tropism	Actions
Beishashen 北沙参 (Coastal Glehnia Root)	Sweet and slightly bitter; Slightly cold	Lung and stomach	1. Nourish lung-yin and clear lung heat 2. Tonify the stomach and promote the production of fluids
Baihe 百合 (Lily Bulb)	Sweet; Slightly cold	Lung, heart and stomach	1. Nourish yin and moisten the lung 2. Clear heat from the heart to calm the mind
Maidong 麦冬 (Dwarf Lilyturf Tuber)	Sweet and slightly bitter; Slightly cold	Lung, stomach and heart	1. Nourish yin and promote the production of fluids 2. Moisten the lung 3. Clear heat from the heart
Shihu 石斛 (Dendrobium)	Sweet; Slightly cold	Stomach and kidney	1. Tonify the stomach and promote the production of fluids 2. Nourish yin and clear asthenic heat
Yuzhu 玉竹 (Solomonseal Rhizome)	Sweet; Slightly cold	Lung and stomach	1. Nourish yin and moisten dryness 2. Promote the production of fluids to quench thirst
Gouqizi 枸杞子 (Wolfberry Seed)	Sweet; Neutral	Liver and kidney	1. Nourish and tonify the kidney and liver 2. Tonify essence and improve vision
Guijia 龟甲 (Tortoise Shell)	Sweet and salty; Cold	Liver, kidney and heart	1. Nourish yin and suppress yang 2. Tonify kidney and strengthen bone 3. Nourish blood and tonify the heart
Heizhima 黑芝麻 (Black Sesame Seed)	Sweet; Neutral	Liver, kidney and large intestine	1. Tonify the kidney and liver 2. Moisten the large intestine 3. Tonify essence and blood

Astringent Herbs 收涩药

Name of Herb	Flavour and Nature	Meridian Tropism	Actions
Wuweizi 五味子 (Chinese Magnoliavine Fruit)	Sour and sweet; Slightly warm	Lung, heart and kidney	1. Reduce sweating 2. Calm the mind 3. Tonify the kidney 4. Tonify qi and promote the production of fluids
Lianzi 莲子 (Lotus seed)	Sweet and astringent; Neutral	Spleen, heart and kidney	1. Prevent abnormal discharge and involuntary seminal emission 2. Tonify the spleen to relieve diarrhoea 3. Tonify the kidney 4. Calm the mind by nourishing the heart

Common Chinese Prescriptions

The prescriptions listed below are representative of the various formulations categorised by their principal therapeutic functions. The Chinese names are provided and, where commonly used, the English translations as well. Each prescription typically ends with 'san' if it is usually prepared as a powder, 'yin' or 'tang' if it is a decoction and 'wan' if in pill form. In practice, most decoctions are also available in pharmacies in the form of pills, tablets or capsules as these are more convenient for daily use.

Diaphoretic Prescriptions		
1	Yinqiaosan 银翘散	Expels wind-heat exogenous pathogens. Eliminates heat and toxins. Often used in the early stage of an external syndrome invaded by wind-heat pathogens.
2	Guizhitang 桂枝汤	Expels wind-cold exogenous pathogens. Regulates the nutrient and defensive qi to strengthen the body. Can be used for treating external syndromes caused by wind-cold exogenous pathogens or for individuals who feel weak and are recovering from chronic illnesses.
Prescriptions for Clearing Internal Heat		
3	Daochisan 导赤散	Clears heat from the heart. Promotes diuresis and nourishes yin. Treats the syndrome of exuberance of heart fire.
4	Longdan Xiegan Tang 龙胆泻肝汤	Purges fire from the liver and gall bladder. Clears dampness and heat in the lower energiser. Treats sthenic syndrome of the exuberance of liver fire.
5	Yunujian 玉女煎	Clears heat from the stomach and nourishes kidney-yin. Treats the syndrome of stomach fire with yin deficiency.

(*Continued*)

(*Continued*)

**Prescriptions for Removing Dampness**		
6	Huoxiang Zhengqi San 藿香正气散	Removes dampness and regulates qi in the abdomen region. Used for treating vomiting and diarrhoea caused by cold dampness and wind.
7	Wulingsan 五苓散	Promotes diuresis and removes dampness. Warms yang-qi to enhance the function of qi to regulate water metabolism. Can be used for treating edema due to retention of water and dampness.
**Prescriptions for Removing Wind-Dampness**		
8	Duhuo Jisheng Tang 独活寄生汤	Expels wind-dampness to relieve arthritic pain. Tonifies kidney, liver, qi and blood. Treats deficiency syndrome in liver, kidney, qi and blood.
9	Danggui Niantong Tang 当归拈痛汤	Drains dampness and clears heat. Expels wind to relieve arthritic pain. Treats damp-heat syndrome.
10	Juanbitang 蠲痹汤	Tonifies qi and nourishes blood. Expels wind and dampness. Treats wind-cold-dampness syndrome and relieves arthritic pain.
**Prescriptions for Promoting Digestion**		
11	Baohewan 保和丸 'Pill for Preserving Harmony'	Promotes digestion of food. Treats food retention syndrome.
**Prescriptions for Promoting Blood Flow and Removing Blood Stasis**		
12	Xuefu Zhuyu Tang 血府逐瘀汤	Promotes blood flow and removes stasis. Regulates qi and relieves pain. Often used for treating blood stasis syndrome.
**Prescriptions for Resolving Phlegm and Relieving Cough**		
13	Qingqi Huatan Tang 清气化痰汤	Clears heat and resolves phlegm. Regulates qi and relieves cough. Treats heat-phlegm syndrome.
14	Banxia Houpo Tang 半夏厚朴汤	Regulates qi to disperse clumps. Suppresses adverse rise of qi and resolves phlegm. Treats 梅核气 *meiheqi* — a feeling of something in the throat that cannot be swallowed or expectorated.
15	Erchen Tang 二陈汤	Removes dampness, resolves phlegm and promotes qi flow. Used in wet cough due to phlegm-dampness with white sputum.

(Continued)

Prescriptions for Calming the Mind		
16	Suanzaoren Tang 酸枣仁汤 'Jujube Seed Decoction'	Nourishes blood and calms the mind. Clears asthenic heat to relieve vexation. Often used to treat insomnia resulting from the deficiency syndrome in liver blood.
17	Tianwang Buxin Dan 天王补心丹	Nourishes yin and blood. Tranquilises heart to calm the mind. Treats yin deficiency syndrome in the heart and kidney.
Prescriptions for Regulating the Liver and Spleen		
18	Xiaoyao San 逍遥散 'Ease Powder'	Soothes the liver and regulates the spleen. Used in stagnation of liver-qi and deficiency of blood and spleen, with liver suppressing spleen (over-restraint relationship).
19	Danzhi Xiaoyaosan 丹栀逍遥散 (extension of ease powder)	Soothes the liver, regulates qi and clears liver fire. Used in liver stagnation stirring up fire.
Prescriptions for Removing Wind (Both Exogenous and Endogenous Wind)		
20	Tianma Gouteng Yin 天麻钩藤饮	Calms the liver to remove endogenous wind. Clears heat and nourishes liver/kidney. Used for treating headache and dizziness caused by hyperactivity of liver-yang syndrome.
21	Xiaofengsan 消风散	Expels wind and nourishes blood. Clears heat and removes dampness. Treats eczema and rubella caused by wind-heat or wind-dampness syndrome.
Prescriptions for Removing Dryness		
22	Qingzao Jiufei Tang 清燥救肺汤	Clears exogenous dry-heat pathogen and moistens the lung. Treats severe syndrome of dryness in the lung.
23	Baihe Gujing Tang 百合固金汤	Nourishes yin and moistens lung. Resolves phlegm and relieves cough. Treats cough caused by the deficiency syndrome of kidney and lung-yin. (Used in the more advanced stage as the lung-yin has been severely damaged.)

(Continued)

(Continued)

	Prescriptions for Tonifying *Qi*	
24	Decoction of the Four Noble Herbs (Sijunzi Tang) 四君子汤	Tonifies qi and strengthens spleen. Used in deficiency syndrome of spleen and stomach.
25	Decoction of the Six Noble Herbs 六君子汤 (extension of Decoction of the Four Noble Herbs)	Used for deficiency of spleen/stomach syndrome with dampness and phlegm.
26	Decoction of *Xiangsha Liujunzi Tang* 香砂六君子汤 (extension of Decoction of Six Noble Herbs)	Used for spleen-stomach deficiency with more pronounced dampness and phlegm leading to qi stagnation.
27	Shenling Baizhu San 参苓白术散	Tonifies qi and strengthens spleen. Resolves dampness. Treats qi deficiency syndrome of the spleen and stomach with dampness.
28	Buzhong Yiqi Tang 补中益气汤	Tonifies qi and strengthens spleen. Uplifts spleen yang-qi. Treats qi deficiency syndrome of the spleen and stomach.
29	Yupingfeng San 玉屏风散 (Jade Screen Powder)	Replenishes qi, consolidates the superficies and arrests perspiration (reduces sweating). Used in individuals with qi deficiency (defensive qi).
30	Pulse-activating Powder 生脉饮 (*Shengmai* Yin)	Tonifies qi and promotes the production of fluids. Astringes yin and arrests sweating. For treatment of deficiency syndrome of qi and yin resulting in spontaneous sweating and chronic dry cough accompanied by breathlessness, fatigue, etc.
	Prescriptions for Tonifying Blood	
31	Decoction of the Four Ingredients 四物汤 (*Siwu Tang*)	Nourishes and regulates blood without introducing stasis. Used in blood deficiency syndrome; Often used for regulating menstruation.
32	Decoction of *Taohong Siwu Tang* 桃红四物汤 (extension of decoction of the four ingredients)	Promotes blood circulation and removes stasis. Used in blood deficiency syndrome with stasis resulting in early menses with blood clots.

(Continued)

33	Chinese Angelica Decoction for Tonifying the Blood 当归补血汤 (Danggui Buxue Tang)	Invigorates qi to promote blood production. Used in blood deficiency syndrome, particularly blood deficiency with fever and headache following childbirth or menstrual disorder with severe loss of blood; anemia.
34	Decoction for Restoring the Spleen 归脾汤 (*Guipitang*)	Tonifies qi and blood. Strengthens the spleen and nourishes the heart. Treats deficiency syndrome in heart and spleen.
35	Danggui Yinzi 当归饮子	Nourishes blood and promotes its flow. Expels wind to relieve pain. Treats eczema or rubella caused by blood deficiency syndrome (with the invasion of wind pathogen).
	Prescriptions for Tonifying *Qi* and Blood	
36	Decoction of the 8 Precious Ingredients 八珍汤	Nourishes qi and blood. Used for those with prolonged weakness of qi and blood caused by excessive haemorrhage and low qi level.
37	Shiquan Dabutang 十全大补汤 'Decoction of 10 Powerful Herbs' (extension of decoction of the 8 precious ingredients)	Warms and tonifies qi and blood. Used in deficiency syndrome in qi and blood, accompanied by slight yang deficiency.
	Prescriptions for Tonifying Yang	
38	Pill for Nourishing Kidney-Yang (Shenqi Wan) 肾气丸	Warms and invigorates kidney-yang. Used to treat deficiency of kidney-yang syndrome, often accompanied by weakness of back and knees, coldness in lower trunk, frequent night urination, sexual dysfunction.
39	Jisheng Shenqi Wan 济生肾气丸 (extension of Shenqi Wan)	Warms kidney-yang and promotes diuresis to relieve edema. It is often used to treat water retention due to kidney-yang deficiency.
	Prescriptions for Tonifying Yin	
40	Liuwei Dihuang Wan 六味地黄丸 'Pill of Six Ingredients with Rehmanniae'	Nourishes yin and invigorates the kidney. Used in deficiency syndrome of kidney and liver-yin, leading to flare up of kidney deficiency fire. Marked by tinnitus, night sweats, emissions, sore throat. Some diabetes patients exhibit such a syndrome.

Annex 3

Glossary of Common Names of Herbs

Chinese Name	中文名	Common Name in English
		A
Aiye	艾叶	Argy wormwood leaf
		B
Baibiandou	白扁豆	White hyacinth bean
Baibu	百部	Stemona root
Baifan	白矾	Alum
Baifuzi	白附子	White aconite root
Baihe	百合	Lily bulb
Baiji	白及	Common bletilla tuber
Baimuer	白木耳	White fungus
Baishao	白芍	White peony root
Baixianpi	白鲜皮	Densefruit pittany root-bark
Baizhi	白芷	Dahurian angelica root
Baizhu	白术	Largehead atractylodes rhizome
Baiziren	柏子仁	Chinese arborvitae kernel
Bajitian	巴戟天	Morinda root
Banlangen	板蓝根	Isatis root
Banxia	半夏	Pinellia tuber
Beishashen	北沙参	Coastal glehnia root
Bingpian	冰片	Bomeol
Binlang	槟榔	Areca seed
Bohe	薄荷	Peppermint
Buguzhi	补骨脂	Malaytea scurfpea fruit

(*Continued*)

(*Continued*)

Chinese Name	中文名	Common Name in English
	C	
Cangerzi	苍耳子	Siberian cocklebur fruit
Cangzhu	苍术	Atractylodes rhizome
Caowu	草乌	Kusnezoff monkshood root
Cebaiye	侧柏叶	Chinese arborvitac twig and leaf
Chaihu	柴胡	Chinese thorowax root
Chantui	蝉蜕	Cicada slough
Chenpi	陈皮	Dried tangerine peel
Chenxiang	沉香	Chinese eaglewood
Cheqianzi	车前子	Plantain seed
Chishao	赤芍	Red peony root
Chishizhi	赤石脂	Red halloysite
Chixiaodou	赤小豆	Red beans
Chuanbeimu	川贝母	Bulb of tendrilleaf fritillary
Chuaniuxi	川牛膝	Medicinal cyathula root
Chuanlianzi	川楝子	Sichuan chinaberry fruit
Chuanshanjia	穿山甲	Pangolin scale
Chuanwu	川乌	Common monkshood mother root
Chuanxiong	川芎	Sichuan lovage root
	D	
Dafupi	大腹皮	Areca peel
Dahuang	大黄	Rhubarb
Danggui	当归	Chinese angelica root
Dangshen	党参	Codonopsis root
Dannanxing	胆南星	Bile arisaema
Danshen	丹参	Red sage root
Daqingye	大青叶	Dyers woad leaf
Dazao	大枣	Chinese date
Dazhuye	淡竹叶	Lophathrum herb
Difuzi	地肤子	Belvedere fruit

(*Continued*)

Chinese Name	中文名	Common Name in English
Digupi	地骨皮	Chinese wolfberry root-bark
Dihuang	地黄	Rehmannia root
Dilong	地龙	Earthworm
Diyu	地榆	Garden burnet root
Doukou	白豆蔻	White cardamon fruit
Duhuo	独活	Doubleteeth pubescent angelica root
Duzhong	杜仲	Eucommia bark
	E	
Ejiao	阿胶	Gelatin
Ezhu	莪术	Zedoray rhizome
	F	
Fabanxia	法半夏	Pinellia tuber processed with radix glycyrrhizae and lime
Fangfeng	防风	Divaricate saposhnikvia root
Fangji	防己	Fourstamen stephania root
Fengfang	蜂房	Honeycomb
Foshou	佛手	Finger citron
Fuling	茯苓	Poria
Fupenzi	覆盆子	Chinese raspberry
Fuxiaomai	浮小麦	Unripe wheat grain
	G	
Gancao	甘草	Liquorice root
Ganjiang	干姜	Dried ginger
Gaolishen	高丽参	Korean ginseng
Gegen	葛根	Kudzuvine root
Gouqizi	枸杞子	Wolfberry
Gouteng	钩藤	Gambir plant
Gualou	瓜蒌	Snake gourd fruit

(*Continued*)

(Continued)

Chinese Name	中文名	Common Name in English
Guijia	龟甲	Tortoise shell
Guizhi	桂枝	Cassia twig
Guya	谷芽	Millet sprout
	H	
Haipiaoxiao	海螵蛸	Cuttlebone
Hanliancao	旱莲草	Eclipta/Yerbadetajo herb
Hehuanhua	合欢花	Albizia flower
Hehuanpi	合欢皮	Silktree albizia bark
Heimuer	黑木耳	Black fungus
Heshouwu	何首乌	Root of Tuber Fleeceflower
Heye	荷叶	Lotus leaf
Honghua	红花	Safflower
Houpo	厚朴	Officinal magnolia bark
Huaijiao	槐角	Japanese pagodatree pod
Huajiao	花椒	Prickly ash peel
Huangbai	黄柏	Amur cork-tree
Huangjing	黄精	Solomonseal rhizome
Huanglian	黄连	Golden thread
Huangqi	黄芪	Astragalus
Huangqin	黄芩	Baical skullcap root
Huashi	滑石	Talc
Huhuanglian	胡黄连	Figwortflower picrorhiza rhizome
Huoxiang	藿香	Cablin patchouli herb
Huzhang	虎杖	Giant Knotweed rhizome
	J	
Jiegeng	桔梗	Platycodon root
Jili	蒺藜	Puncturevine caltrop fruit
Jineijin	鸡内金	Chicken's gizzard skin
Jingjie	荆芥	Fineleaf schizonepeta herb

(*Continued*)

Chinese Name	中文名	Common Name in English
Jinmaogouji	金毛狗脊	Chain fern rhizome
Jinzhencai	金针菜	Dried Lily flower
Jixueteng	鸡血藤	Suberect spatholobus stem
Juhong	橘红	Red tangerine peel
Juhua	菊花	Chrysanthemum flower
Juiyinhua	金银花	Honeysuckle flower
	K	
Kuandonghua	款冬花	Common coltsfoot flower
Kushen	苦参	Lightyellow sophora root
Kuxingren	苦杏仁	Bitter apricot seed
	L	
Lianqiao	连翘	Weeping forsythia gapsule
Lianzi	莲子	Lotus seed
Longdancao	龙胆草	Chinese gentian
Longyanrou	龙眼肉	Longan aril
Luhui	芦荟	Aloes
Lulutong	路路通	Sweet gum fruit
	M	
Machixian	马齿苋	Purslane herb
Mahuang	麻黄	Ephedra
Maidong	麦冬	Dwarf lilyturf tuber
Maiya	麦芽	Germinated barley
Mingdangshen	明党参	Medicinal changium root
Mudanpi	牡丹皮	Tree peony bark
Muli	牡蛎	Oyster shell
Muxiang	木香	Costus root
	N	
Niubangzi	牛蒡子	Burdock seed
Niuxi	牛膝	Two tooth achyranthes root
Nvzhenzi	女贞子	Glossy privet fruit

(*Continued*)

(*Continued*)

Chinese Name	中文名	Common Name in English
	P	
Peilan	佩兰	Fortune eupatorium herb
Pipaye	枇杷叶	Loquat leaf
Pugongying	蒲公英	Dandelion
Puhuang	蒲黄	Cattail pollen
	Q	
Qiancao	茜草	India madder root
Qianghuo	羌活	Incised notoptergium rhizome
Qianniuzi	牵牛子	Pharbitis seed
Qianshi	芡实	Gordon seed
Qingdai	青黛	Natural indigo
Qinghao	青蒿	Sweet wormwood herb
Qingpi	青皮	Green tangerine peel
Qinjiao	秦艽	Largeleaf gentian root
Quanxie	全蝎	Scorpion
	R	
Rendongteng	忍冬藤	Honeysuckle stem
Renshen	人参	Ginseng
Roucongrong	肉苁蓉	Desertliving cistanche
Rougui	肉桂	Cassia bark
	S	
Sangbaipi	桑白皮	White mulberry root-bark
Sangjisheng	桑寄生	Chinese taxillus herb/Mulberry mistletoe stems
Sangshen	桑椹	Mulberry fruit
Sangye	桑叶	Mulberry leaf
Sanleng	三棱	Common burreed tuber
Sanqi	三七	Panax notoginseng
Shanyao	山药	Chinese yam
Shanzha	山楂	Hawthorn fruit
Shanzhuyu	山茱萸	Asiatic comelian cherry fruit

(*Continued*)

Chinese Name	中文名	Common Name in English
Sharen	砂仁	Villous amomum fruit
Shegan	射干	Blackberry lily rhizome
Shejiang	生姜	Fresh ginger
Shengma	升麻	Large trifoliolious bugbane rhizome
Shenjincao	伸筋草	Common club moss
Shichangpu	石菖蒲	Grassleaf sweetflag rhizome
Shigao	石膏	Gypsum
Shihu	石斛	Dendrobium
Shijunzi	使君子	Rangooncreeper fruit
Shudihuang	熟地黄	Processed rehmannia root
Shuizhi	水蛭	Leech
Sigua	丝瓜	Loofah
Suanzaoren	酸枣仁	Spine date seed
Sumu	苏木	Sappan wood
Suzi	苏子	Perilla fruit
	T	
Taizishen	太子参	Heterophylly false starwort root
Taoren	桃仁	Peach seed
Tianhuafen	天花粉	Snakegourd root
Tianma	天麻	Tall gastrodia tuber
Tinglizi	葶苈子	Pepperweed seed
Tongcao	通草	Ricepaperplant pith
Tufuling	土茯苓	Glabrous greenbrier rhizome
Tusizi	菟丝子	Dodder seed
	W	
Wangbuliuxing	王不留行	Cowberb seed
Wugong	蜈蚣	Centipede
Wujiai	五加皮	Slenderstyle acanthopanax bark
Wumei	乌梅	Smoked plum
Wuweizi	五味子	Chinese magnolia vine fruit
Wuyao	乌药	Combined spicebush root

(*Continued*)

(Continued)

Chinese Name	中文名	Common Name in English
Wuzhuyu	吴茱萸	Medicinal evodia fruit
		X
Xiakucao	夏枯草	Common selfheal fruit-spike
Xiangfu	香附	Nutgrass galingale rhizome
Xiangru	香薷	Mosia herb
Xianhecao	仙鹤草	Hairyvein agrimonia herb
Xianmao	仙茅	Common curculigo rhizome
Xiebai	薤白	Long-stamen onion bulb
Xinyi	辛夷	Biond magnolia flower
Xixin	细辛	Manchurian wildginger
Xuanfuhua	旋复花	Inula flower
Xuanshen	玄参	Figwort root
Xuchangqing	徐长卿	Paniculate swallowwort root
Xuduan	续断	Himalayan teasel root
Xueyutan	血余炭	Carbonised hair
		Y
Yanhusuo	延胡索	Rhizoma corydalis/Corydalis tuber
Yejuhua	野菊花	Wild chrysanthemum flower
Yimucao	益母草	Motherwort herb
Yinchaihu	银柴胡	Starwort root
Yinchen	茵陈	Virgate wormwood herb
Yinyanghuo	淫羊藿	Epimedium herb
Yiyiren	薏苡仁	Job's tears/Chinese Barley
Yuanzhi	远志	Thinleaf milkwort root
Yujin	郁金	Tumeric root tuber
Yuxingcao	鱼腥草	Heartleaf houttuynia herb
Yuzhu	玉竹	Solomonseal rhizome
		Z
Zelan	泽兰	Hirsute shiny bugleweed herb
Zexie	泽泻	Oriental waterplantain rhizome
Zhebeimu	浙贝母	Bulb of Thungberg fritillary

(*Continued*)

Chinese Name	中文名	Common Name in English
Zhenzhumu	珍珠母	Nacre
Zhifuzi	制附子	Prepared common monkshood daughter root
Zhigancao	炙甘草	Liquorice root processed with honey
Zhimu	知母	Common anemarrhena rhizome
Zhiqiao	枳壳	Orange fruit
Zhishi	枳实	Immature orange fruit
Zhizi	栀子	Cape jasmine fruit
Zhuling	猪苓	Polyporus umbellatus
Zhuru	竹茹	Bamboo shavings
Zicao	紫草	Arnebia root
Zisugeng	紫苏梗	Perilla stem
Zisuye	紫苏叶	Perilla leaf

References

Abrass, IB (1990) The biology and physiology of ageing. *The Western Journal of Medicine*, 153(6): 641–645.

Benson H and Klipper MZ (1975). *The Relaxation Response*. Mass Market Paperback.

Buettner, D (2008) *The Blue Zones*. Washington: National Geographic.

Cleveland Clinic (2022) Chinese Herbal Therapy. https://my.clevelandclinic. org/departments/wellness/integrative/treatments-services/chinese-herbal-therapy Retrieved 5th March 2022

Drake Inner Prizes.com/Energy Medicine (2022). Retrieved 13th May 2022.

Harvard Medical School (2018) "An Introduction to Tai Chi," *Harvard Health Publishing*, p3.

Hewlings, SJ and Kalman, DS (2017) Curcumin: A Review of Its Effects on Human Health. https://www.ncbi.nlm.nih.gov/pmc/articles/ PMC5664031/ Retrieved 9th May 2022

Hong, H (2013) *Acupuncture: Theories and Evidence*. World Scientific Publishing Company.

Hong, H (2016) *Principles of Chinese Medicine: A Modern Interpretation*. London: Imperial College Press.

Hong, H (2017) "Can Chinese Medicine and Biomedicine Converge?" *Asia-Pacific Biotech News* (March 2017) Vol 21. No 3

Hong, H (2020) *The Rule of Culture: Corporate and State Governance in China and East Asia*. London: Routledge

Ilardi, S (2013) Depression as a disease of civilization, TED talk May 2013. https://www.youtube.com/watch?v=drv3BP0Fdi8 Retrieved 6th May 2022.

Jinpa T (2015) *A Fearless Heart*. London: Piatkus (Little, Brown Book Group).

Le Fanu, J (2011) *The Rise and Fall of Modern Medicine*. New York: Hachette Digital.

Life in the Fastlane (2022) Oslerisms. https://litfl.com/eponymictionary/oslerisms/ Retrieved 7th March, 2022

Liu, Z and Ma, L (2007) *Health Preservation of TCM*, Renmin Medical Publishing, p.315–6

Longhurst, JC (2010). Defining Meridians: A Modern Basis of Understanding. *Journal of Acupuncture and Meridian Studies*. Vol 3, Issue 2, Pg 67–74

Myn Lyu *et al* (2021) Traditional Chinese medicine in Covid-19. *Science Direct*, Nov 2021. https://www.sciencedirect.com/science/article/pii/S2211383521003506 Retrieved 5th March,2202.

Needham J (2016) *Science and Civilisation in China*, Vol VI, Part VI. Cambridge University Press.

Nobel Prize in Physiology or Medicine (2017) Press release https://www.nobelprize.org/prizes/medicine/2017/press-release/ Retrieved 15th May 2022

Oxford (2007) *Oxford Concise Medical Dictionary* (2007) 4th Edition. Oxford: Oxford University Press.

Rawlins, MD (16 October 2008). On the Evidence for Decisions about the Use of Therapeutic Interventions. Harvein Oration, Royal College of Physicians.

Sinclair, D A (2019) *Lifespan*, Atria Books.

Sun *et al* (2021) Health benefits of wolfberry (Gou Qi Zi, Fructus barbarum L.) on the basis of ancient Chinese herbalism and Western modern medicine. *Avicenna J Phytomed*, Mar-Apr 2021; 11(2): 109–119.

Wachtel-Galor, S *et al* (2011) Ganoderma lucidum (Lingzhi or Reishi): A Medicinal Mushroom. Based on *Herbal Medicine: Biomolecular and Clinical Aspects*. 2nd edition, Chapter 9. Taylor and Francis. Presented in National Library of Medicine. https://www.ncbi.nlm.nih.gov/books/NBK92757/ Retrieved 9th May 2022.

Weil, A (1995) *Natural Health, Natural Medicine*. Houghton Mifflin William Osler Quotes. http://www.brainyquote.com/quotes/authors/w/william_osler.html Retrieved 8 September 2016).

Wittie, W (2018) Nixon and Scheel in China: Acupuncture and Anesthesia in East and West Germany. https://www.anesthesiahistoryjournal.org/article/S2352-4529(17)30158-5/references Retrieved 13th May 2022

World Health Organisation (2004) Report of the International Expert Meeting to review and analyse clinical reports on combination treatment for SARS (2004).

World Health Organization (2015). Opening Remarks at the International Forum on Traditional Medicine, China, Macao SAR, 19th August 2015. http://who.int/dg/speeches/2015/traditional-medicine/en/ Retrieved 12th Sept 2016.

Worrall, L (2002) What evidence in evidence-based medicine? *Philosophy of Science*, 69:316–330.

Wu Changguo (2002) *Basic Theory of Traditional Chinese Medicine*, Publishing House of Shanghai University of Traditional Chinese Medicine, 2002. https://apps.who.int/iris/handle/10665/43029 Retrieved 5th March, 2022

黄海 (2021)《中医基础学新释》，北京求真出版社

谢梦洲 (主编) (2016)中医药膳学 (第九版)，中国中医药出版社

Index

Additional information on TCM

Readers may find following websites and video links helpful for expanding their knowledge of TCM.

1. Website of Renhai Centre Limited www.renhai.com.sg. See "Resources".
2. C3A portal www.c3a.org.sg/WatchVideo
3. Stephen Ilardi on "Disease of Civilization" www.youtube.com/watch?v=drv3BP0Fdi8
4. Dan Buettner on the Blue Zones www.youtube.com/watch?v=3GfXNk-MiHg
5. Hong Hai on Yangsheng:
   Part 1: https://www.youtube.com/watch?v=nZesRVdR4YQ
   Part 2: https://www.youtube.com/watch?v=syvTOzA2w-o

Printed in the United States
by Baker & Taylor Publisher Services